NURSING INFORMATICS

A COMPREHENSIVE GUIDE TO DIGITAL HEALTH CARE TRENDS TOOLS AND PRACTICES

JASON MILLICAN

Copyright © 2024 JASON MILLICAN

All rights reserved

The characters and events portrayed in this book are fictitious. Any similarity to real persons, living or dead, is coincidental and not intended by the author.

No part of this book may be reproduced, or stored in a retrieval system, or transmitted in any form or by any means, electronic, mechanical, photocopying, recording, or otherwise, without express written permission of the publisher.

CONTENTS

Title Page
Copyright
CHAPTER ONE — 1
CHAPTER TWO — 18
CHAPTER THREE — 41
CHAPTER FOUR — 52
CHAPTER FIVE — 64
CHAPTER SIX — 76
CHAPTER SEVEN — 90

INTRODUCTION

The way nursing care is administered and provided in the current healthcare environment has completely changed as a result of technology integration. Nursing informatics, a specialty area that blends nursing science with information management and technology, is essential to this shift. The definition and application of nursing informatics will be examined in this book, along with its importance, fundamental ideas, and contribution to better patient outcomes and healthcare delivery.

In order to discover, define, manage, and transmit data, information, knowledge, and wisdom in nursing practice, the specialty of nursing informatics blends nursing science with information management and analytical sciences. It includes all applications of information and communication technology to nursing practice, teaching, research, and administration. Fundamentally, the goal of nursing informatics is to maximize the use of technology and information systems to improve the efficacy, safety, and quality of nursing care.

Improving clinical practice is one of nursing informatics' main goals. This entails supporting evidence-based practice, expediting documentation, and facilitating provider communication through the use of clinical decision support systems (CDSS), electronic health records (EHRs), and other health information technologies. Nurses can make educated judgments and provide individualized care by using informatics technologies to gather, store, and analyze patient data.

By teaching nurses how to use technology in their practice, nursing informatics broadens its scope to include education and training. It entails teaching nursing students digital literacy, giving them practical instruction on electronic documentation systems, and incorporating informatics abilities into nursing courses. Through the use of informatics education, nurses can contribute to the growth of healthcare technology by gaining the skills necessary to navigate complicated health information systems.

The application of nursing informatics to research and evidence-based practice is a noteworthy additional feature. With the use of informatics tools, nurses can more easily gather, analyze, and disseminate data, conduct research studies, assess interventions, and provide evidence to enhance patient outcomes. Nurses can use informatics to access large databases of medical information, do complex data analysis, and help create clinical guidelines and best practices.

In healthcare leadership and administration, nursing informatics is also very important. The design, implementation, and evaluation of information systems that support administrative tasks including scheduling, resource allocation, and performance monitoring are carried out by nurse informaticists in collaboration with interdisciplinary teams. Additionally, at the corporate and governmental levels, informatics proficiency is crucial for policy formation, strategic planning, and decision-making procedures.

Nursing informatics' primary concerns are patient safety and quality improvement. Nurses can spot patterns, trends, and opportunities for enhancement in patient care procedures by utilizing technology and data analytics. With the use of informatics technologies, nurses may monitor patient outcomes, adverse events, and medication errors in real time. This allows them to conduct interventions that improve safety, reduce errors, and maximize the quality of care they provide.

By bridging the gap between technology, other healthcare fields, and nursing practice, nursing informatics fosters interdisciplinary collaboration. In order to create and execute integrated information systems that satisfy the many demands of healthcare stakeholders, nurse informaticists work in conjunction with IT specialists, physicians, administrators, and legislators. Nursing informatics stimulates creativity, encourages communication, and makes it easier for information to be seamlessly shared across healthcare settings through multidisciplinary teamwork.

Nursing practice, education, research, and administration are all greatly advanced by the dynamic and varied profession of nursing informatics. Its scope includes a wide range of initiatives meant to maximize the potential of information systems and technology to improve clinical workflows, patient outcomes, and healthcare delivery quality and safety. Nursing informatics is going to be at the forefront as technology develops and changes the healthcare environment because it helps nurses understand the intricacies of contemporary healthcare and provide high-quality, patient-centered care.

Benefits of Nursing Informatics

The fusion of nursing science, information management, and technology—known as nursing informatics—offers numerous advantages in the fields of administration, research, teaching, and healthcare delivery.

By giving nurses access to timely and accurate information, nursing informatics improves the standard and security of patient care. Healthcare providers can more easily maintain continuity of care and coordinate patient treatment thanks to electronic health records (EHRs), which allow for thorough documentation of patient assessments, actions, and outcomes. Better patient outcomes are ultimately achieved when nurses use clinical decision support systems (CDSS) to help them make evidence-based judgments, lower medication errors, and prevent adverse events.

Nursing informatics increases productivity and efficiency in healthcare environments by automating repetitive processes and optimizing clinical workflows. By doing away with the necessity for manual charting, electronic documentation solutions minimize paperwork and documentation time. Accurate dosing and delivery of medications is ensured via barcode scanning and drug administration systems, which enhance medication management procedures. Informatics tools also make it easier for interdisciplinary teams to collaborate and communicate in real time, which promotes effective resource management and care coordination.

With the ability to access the most recent research findings, clinical recommendations, and best practices, nursing informatics plays a vital role in advancing evidence-based practice (EBP) among nurses. In order to enable nurses to provide care that is founded on the best available evidence, information systems facilitate the integration of evidence into clinical decision-making procedures. Furthermore, nurses are better equipped to conduct research studies, assess interventions, and contribute to the creation of new knowledge in nursing practice because of informatics technologies that make data collecting, analysis, and distribution easier.

Patients are empowered to actively participate in their care and self-management through the use of informatics technologies including patient portals, mobile health apps, and telehealth platforms. Through digital platforms, patients can contact with healthcare practitioners, access their health records, make appointments, and receive educational resources. Nursing informatics improves patient happiness, adherence to treatment programs, and health outcomes by encouraging patient engagement and self-care.

Throughout the healthcare continuum, nursing informatics promotes communication and cooperation between patients, healthcare providers, and other stakeholders. The utilization of electronic communication technologies facilitates safe messaging, virtual consultations, and remote monitoring, thereby removing geographical constraints and allowing prompt access to healthcare services. Additionally, by offering a common platform for exchanging patient data, organizing care plans, and monitoring patient advancement, informatics solutions facilitate interdisciplinary collaboration and enhance care coordination as well as patient outcomes.

Nurses may now gather, evaluate, and understand vast amounts of data to find trends, patterns, and places where patient care procedures need to be improved thanks to informatics technologies. In order to enhance quality and safety, data analytics tools like machine learning, predictive modeling, and data visualization enable nurses to make data-driven decisions, allocate resources optimally, and carry out focused interventions. Furthermore, healthcare organizations can identify areas for development and track progress over time by using informatics technologies to facilitate performance monitoring, benchmarking, and outcomes measurement.

Nursing informatics allows nurses to stay up to date with technological and informatics practice improvements by providing chances for professional growth and lifetime learning. Nursing curricula and continuing education programs incorporate informatics capabilities, giving nurses the knowledge and abilities they need to apply informatics technologies in their practice. For nurses interested in a career in informatics, professional associations and nursing informatics certification programs also provide networking opportunities, tools, and support.

Current Trends in Nursing Informatics

The COVID-19 pandemic hastened the use of remote monitoring and telehealth in nursing practice and other healthcare settings. Nurses can monitor patients remotely, conduct virtual consultations, and administer follow-up care from a distance thanks to telehealth platforms. This trend is anticipated to continue as more healthcare institutions adopt telehealth, which they view as an affordable and practical means of providing care, especially for patients who live in underserved or rural locations.

In order to streamline regular processes, evaluate massive information, and enhance clinical decision-making, AI and machine learning technologies are being progressively incorporated into nursing informatics. Clinical decision support systems (CDSS) with AI capabilities can assist nurses in finding trends, forecasting results, and customizing treatment regimens based on patient data. As artificial intelligence (AI) develops, nurses will be essential in utilizing these tools to improve patient outcomes and care.

Numerous wearable technologies, health monitoring applications, and electronic health records (EHRs) have led to the daily generation of enormous volumes of healthcare data. Nurses can use big data analytics tools to monitor population health, spot patterns, and enhance care delivery procedures. Nurses can improve the effectiveness and efficiency of care delivery by using big data to get useful insights about patient populations, disease patterns, and healthcare utilization.

Both patients and healthcare professionals are finding greater and greater use of mobile health applications. With the help of these apps, patients may use their smartphones or tablets to monitor their health indicators, interact with their care team, and access instructional materials. By encouraging patient participation, assisting with self-management, and offering remote monitoring and assistance, nurses can use mHealth apps to enhance patient outcomes and satisfaction.

Challenges in Nursing Informatics

Interoperability, or the capacity of various information systems and devices to interchange and use data seamlessly, is one of the main issues in nursing informatics. Healthcare companies frequently utilize a variety of IT systems, some of which may not be able to connect with one another well, resulting in inconsistent data and inefficient workflows. Standardized data formats, widely used language, and reliable integration solutions—all of which can be difficult and expensive to implement—are necessary to achieve interoperability.

Data security and privacy are becoming more and more of a problem as healthcare data digitizes. Strict laws like the Health Insurance Portability and Accountability Act (HIPAA) must be followed by nurses in order to guarantee the privacy, accuracy, and accessibility of patient data. But there are still incidents of healthcare data breaches, which emphasizes the necessity of strong cybersecurity defenses, personnel education, and data governance structures to shield private patient information from exposure or illegal access.

The difference in access to information and communication technology (ICT) between those with and those without is known as the "digital divide." By preventing underprivileged communities from accessing patient portals, telehealth services, and health information resources, the digital divide in healthcare has the potential to worsen health disparities. It is imperative for nurses to acknowledge and tackle these inequalities by means of advancing digital literacy, granting access to technology, and championing legislation that guarantee fair and equal access to healthcare resources and data.

When implementing new informatics technology, healthcare providers accustomed to paper-based methods may oppose the change and workflows may get disrupted. It might be difficult for nurses to manage workflow changes, get past colleagues' opposition, and adjust to new technology. To guarantee that informatics solutions fit end-user demands and clinical processes, nurses must be included in the design, implementation, and optimization phases.

The field of nursing informatics is rapidly evolving due to the impact of developing technology and shifting healthcare environments. While there are many chances to improve patient care and outcomes with these trends, nurses must also overcome a number of obstacles, including reluctance to change, data security concerns, interoperability issues, and health disparities. Nurses can use technology to improve patient outcomes, nursing practice, and healthcare delivery by proactively addressing these issues and successfully utilizing informatics technologies.

CHAPTER ONE

Information Systems in Healthcare

Information systems are essential to contemporary healthcare because they make it easier to manage, process, and share data and information about health. These systems are made to assist a range of activities in the healthcare process, such as research, clinical decision-making, administrative work, and patient care.

EHR systems are all-inclusive electronic databases that hold patient health data, such as diagnosis, prescriptions, allergies, test results from labs, and treatment regimens. EHRs improve patient safety, decrease medical errors, and improve care coordination by enabling healthcare practitioners to securely access and share patient data. EHRs also aid in quality reporting, order entry, clinical documentation, and decision assistance, supporting evidence-based practice and QI projects.

Healthcare organizations, providers, and stakeholders can exchange patient health information electronically thanks to HIE platforms. Regardless of the platform or vendor, HIEs enable authorized users to easily access and exchange patient data across various health IT systems. HIEs enable population health management, public health reporting, care coordination, and transitions of care by promoting interoperability and data exchange.

Software solutions known as CDSS are designed to improve clinical decision-making at the point of care by giving doctors useful information and suggestions.

In order to provide warnings, reminders, and treatment recommendations that are specific to each patient's unique characteristics and the clinical setting, CDSS analyzes patient data, clinical guidelines, and best practices. By assisting doctors in identifying possible medication errors, harmful drug interactions, and gaps in treatment, these technologies eventually enhance patient outcomes and safety.

Medical imaging data, including X-rays, CT, MRI, and ultrasound scans, are stored, retrieved, and distributed using Picture Archiving and Communication Systems (PACS), which are specialist inform byation systems. PACS eliminates the need for film-based radiography film by enabling healthcare practitioners to electronically store and retrieve digital pictures. PACS systems interface with electronic health records (EHRs) to allow easy access to imaging studies from within the patient's EHR and to promote interdisciplinary collaboration between physicians, radiologists, and other clinicians.

Software platforms called Laboratory Information Systems (LIS) are used to handle test orders, specimen processing, test results, and reporting in laboratories. LIS ensures accuracy and traceability of laboratory data, automates result reporting, and streamlines laboratory procedures. Numerous laboratory disciplines, such as clinical chemistry, hematology, microbiology, and pathology, are supported by these systems. By giving healthcare practitioners fast access to diagnostic data, LIS integration with EHRs facilitates clinical decision-making and allows real-time access to laboratory results.

Specialized information systems called radiography Information Systems (RIS) are used to handle scheduling, reporting, and processes in radiography. Radiology orders, images, and reports can be electronically captured, stored, and distributed with the help of RIS. These technologies facilitate communication between radiologists, technicians, and referring physicians while streamlining radiological operations and increasing workflow efficiency. The smooth coordination of radiology services within the larger healthcare delivery system is made possible by RIS integration with PACS and EHRs.

Pharmacy Information Systems (PIS) are software systems that are used in healthcare organizations to manage various medication-related tasks, such as billing, inventory management, prescription administration, and dispensing. PIS assist with drug usage assessment, prescription processing, medication order entry, and medication reconciliation. These systems improve pharmaceutical safety by giving doctors access to thorough medication profiles, alerts about drug interactions, and dose recommendations based on solid data. The seamless coordination and communication between pharmacies and other healthcare professionals is made possible by PIS integration with EHRs.

Platforms for telehealth and telemedicine make it possible to use telecommunications technology to provide medical care remotely. These platforms facilitate remote monitoring, teleconferencing, teleeducation, and virtual consultations. Telehealth systems lower healthcare inequities, enhance care coordination for patients with chronic diseases, and make care more accessible to patients living in rural or disadvantaged areas. Additionally, these systems facilitate interdisciplinary communication between medical professionals and make it possible to offer specialized services like telepsychiatry, teledermatology, and telestroke treatment.

Information systems are essential tools for modern healthcare organizations, helping them to efficiently digitize, organize, and disseminate health-related data and information. Healthcare providers can improve clinical decision-making, expedite workflows, foster collaboration throughout the healthcare continuum, and improve patient care by utilizing these tools. Information systems will become more and more important as technology develops, influencing how healthcare is delivered in the future and enhancing patient outcomes.

Competencies in nursing informatics

The knowledge, skills, and abilities that nurses require to apply information technology and information management concepts in their practice are included in nursing informatics competencies. In order to effectively negotiate the intricacies of contemporary healthcare delivery, utilize technology to enhance patient care, and promote the specialty of nursing informatics, nurses must possess these competencies.

Effective management of health information, including data collection, documentation, storage, retrieval, and distribution, is a must for nurses. Proficiency in information management involves comprehending vocabulary, classification schemes, data standards, and data integrity, confidentiality, and security principles. Health information exchange (HIE) platforms, electronic health record (EHR) systems, and other informatics tools should enable nurses to precisely and securely collect, organize, and communicate patient data.

A wide range of technological instruments and devices that are frequently utilized in healthcare settings require proficiency from nurses. This entails having command of computers, mobile devices, and other electronic equipment in addition to being acquainted with software programs like telehealth platforms, clinical decision support systems (CDSS), and electronic health record (EHR) systems. To guarantee the efficient and successful use of technology in nursing practice, competencies in technology competence also include comprehension of fundamental troubleshooting techniques, software navigation, and user interface design concepts.

Clinical decision support, which uses technology to deliver evidence-based advice and recommendations at the point of care, is a competency that nurses must acquire. Clinical data interpretation, patient needs assessment, and the incorporation of pertinent clinical guidelines, best practices, and evidence-based resources into clinical decision-making processes are all included in this. To spot possible mistakes, stop unfavorable events, and improve patient outcomes, nurses should be able to utilize CDSS, alerts, reminders, and decision support tools.

The ability to safely share patient information electronically between healthcare organizations, providers, and stakeholders is a competency that nurses must possess. This entails being aware of the privacy laws controlling HIE, data sharing protocols, and interoperability principles. Through the use of HIE platforms, nurses should be able to efficiently manage care transitions, promote care coordination, and access, retrieve, and share patient information across various health IT systems.

In order to inform clinical decision-making and enhance patient outcomes, nurses must be competent in evidence-based practice, which incorporates the use of research findings, clinical expertise, and patient preferences. This involves the capacity to evaluate research literature critically, recognize pertinent evidence, and implement evidence-based protocols and standards in nursing practice. In order to support safe, efficient, and patient-centered care, nurses should be able to use informatics tools to access electronic databases, look up evidence, and incorporate research findings into clinical workflows.

In order to effectively advocate for the use of informatics technologies, foster an innovative culture, and facilitate interdisciplinary teamwork, nurses need to possess competencies in leadership and collaboration. Effective communication skills with coworkers, patients, and stakeholders are all part of this, as are the capacity to manage change, spearhead informatics projects, and create an atmosphere that is conducive to technology adoption. It should be possible for nurses to work with interdisciplinary teams, take part in informatics committees, and influence the creation of informatics standards, policies, and procedures inside their organizations.

To stay up to date with developments in nursing

informatics and guarantee competence in using informatics tools, nurses require competencies in education and training. Participating in continuing education courses, going to informatics conferences, and obtaining informatics qualifications and certificates are all examples of this. In addition, nurses should be competent in teaching and training patients, students, and coworkers in informatics. This includes creating instructional materials, giving presentations, and facilitating practical training.These competences enable nurses to expand nursing informatics as a specialty, improve clinical decision-making, advance evidence-based practice, and improve patient care. Nurses must engage in ongoing education, training, and professional development to maintain and improve their informatics competencies in the always changing healthcare environment.

Nursing informatics capabilities have different educational and training needs based on the particular roles and responsibilities in the profession. Nonetheless, the following broad recommendations for instruction and training exist:

Bachelor of Science in Nursing (BSN): The minimal educational qualification for many nursing informatics roles is a BSN. Nursing informatics positions require a background in nursing science, evidence-based practice, and healthcare delivery, all of which are covered in BSN programs.

Master of Science in Nursing (MSN): Graduate-level education offers specific knowledge and abilities in informatics principles, technology applications, and leadership. An MSN with an emphasis in nursing informatics is one example of this type of advanced education. Research methodologies, data management, healthcare information systems, and informatics theory are all common subjects covered in MSN programs.

Advanced doctoral degrees in nursing, such as the Doctor of Nursing Practice (DNP) or PhD in Nursing, equip nurses for leadership positions in nursing informatics practice, research, and teaching. While PhD programs concentrate on research methodologies, theory development, and academic inquiry, DNP programs emphasize advanced practice skills, quality improvement, and systems leadership.

Taking courses in informatics is crucial if you want to become competent in fields like health information exchange, clinical decision support, technical proficiency, and information management. Basics of health informatics, database administration, clinical decision support systems, and telehealth applications are a few examples of the subjects that may be covered in courses.

In addition to being offered by professional associations, educational institutions, and online learning platforms, informatics training can be finished as part of a nursing degree program.

Applying informatics knowledge and skills in actual healthcare settings requires clinical experience. Through clinical practicums, internships, and on-the-job training, nurses can get practical experience using informatics tools and systems.

Through clinical experience, nurses can advance their knowledge in areas like telehealth applications, clinical decision support systems, health information exchange (HIE), and electronic health records (EHRs).

A certification in nursing informatics shows expertise and ability in the subject, and employers may need it or prefer it for specific positions. For registered nurses with at least two years of expertise in nursing informatics, the American Nurses Credentialing Center (ANCC) offers the Informatics Nursing Certification (RN-BC).

Nursing informatics professionals can also obtain certification programs and credentials from professional associations like the Healthcare Information and Management Systems Society (HIMSS). Examples of these include the Certified Professional in Healthcare Information and Management Systems (CPHIMS) and the Certified Associate in Healthcare Information and Management Systems (CAHIMS).

Since the field of nursing informatics is quickly developing, continuing education and professional development are crucial for being up to date with new developments in technology, informatics concepts, and industry best practices. Nurses can improve their nursing informatics knowledge and abilities by attending conferences, workshops, webinars, and online courses.

Nursing informatics practitioners can benefit from professional associations like the American Nursing Informatics Association (ANIA) and HIMSS, which provide instructional materials, networking opportunities, and professional development activities. Nursing professionals can acquire the information, skills, and abilities required to succeed in nursing informatics roles and significantly impact healthcare informatics practice and research by completing the required education and training.

Certification and Credentialing

In nursing informatics, certification and credentialing are crucial procedures that verify the expertise, proficiencies, and understanding of nurses practicing in the field. These certifications show that a nurse is knowledgeable with healthcare information management, technological applications, and informatics principles.

An optional approach that enables nurses to show their expertise in the field is certification in nursing informatics. Nurses' knowledge, skills, and abilities in a variety of nursing informatics domains, such as clinical decision support, technology proficiency, information management, and health information exchange, are evaluated via certification tests.

The American Nurses Credentialing Center (ANCC) is the main certifying authority for nursing informatics certification. For registered nurses with at least two years of experience in nursing informatics, the ANCC offers the Informatics Nursing Certification (RN-BC). Topics include data management, informatics concepts, healthcare information systems, and regulatory requirements are covered in the test.

The certifying authority has specified specific standards for education and experience that candidates must achieve in order to be eligible for nursing informatics certification. For instance, the ANCC mandates that applicants hold an active, valid RN license, have practiced nursing informatics for at least 2,000 hours during the previous three years, and have completed at least 30 hours of continuing education in the field.

Multiple-choice questions on the nursing informatics certification test evaluate a candidate's knowledge and proficiency in a range of nursing informatics topics. Topics including data management and analytics, technology and information systems, ethical and legal issues, leadership, and professional practice are all covered in the exam. In order to receive certification, candidates need to pass the test.

A nurse's certification in nursing informatics usually has a time limit after which it must be renewed in order to keep their license. Achieving continuing education credits, proving continuous professional development, and satisfying practice hour requirements are a few examples of renewal requirements. In order to prove their ongoing competency, candidates may also be required by certifying bodies to retake the certification exam on a regular basis.

In the field of nursing informatics, credentialing is the process of confirming a nurse's credentials, background, and skill set. Employers may demand or prefer credentialing for specific nursing informatics roles, especially those involving leadership, academia, and research.

Depending on their degree of training, experience, and area of expertise, nursing informatics specialists can hold a variety of credentials. A Master of Science in Nursing (MSN) with a concentration in nursing informatics or a Doctor of Nursing Practice (DNP) with an informatics focus are two common credentials in nursing informatics. Other credentials include Certified Professional in Healthcare Information and Management Systems (CPHIMS), Certified Associate in Healthcare Information and Management Systems (CAHIMS), and various academic degrees.

Associations for professionals like the American Nursing Informatics Association (ANIA),Nursing informatics practitioners can obtain certifications and credentialing programs from the American Medical Informatics Association (AMIA) and the Healthcare Information and Management Systems Society (HIMSS). For nurses looking to grow in nursing informatics, these organizations offer tools, networking opportunities, and assistance.Qq As a requirement for employment, some businesses could favor or demand that nursing informatics professionals possess particular credentials or certificates.

Credentialing may improve a nurse's chances of landing a job and moving up the nursing informatics ladder by demonstrating their dedication to professional growth and ability.

In conclusion, nursing informatics certification and credentialing are important procedures that attest to a nurse's expertise in the subject. While credentialing confirms a nurse's qualifications, certification examinations measure a nurse's skill in specific areas of nursing informatics.In this dynamic and quickly changing sector, nurses can showcase their competence, build their professional reputation, and further their careers by earning certification and qualifications in nursing informatics.

Opportunities for professional growth

In order for nurses to stay current with technological innovations, informatics concepts, and best practices in healthcare delivery, they must have access to professional development opportunities in nursing informatics. By taking advantage of these chances, nurses can improve their nursing informatics knowledge, abilities, and competences, which will help them flourish professionally. In nursing informatics, the following are some typical options for professional development:

Nursing informatics-related courses, conferences, seminars, and webinars are available through continuing education programs. Electronic health records (EHRs), clinical decision support systems (CDSS), data analytics, and telehealth applications are just a few of the topics covered in these programs.

Professional associations, educational institutions, healthcare facilities, and online learning platforms all provide continuing education programs. By taking part in these programs, nurses can obtain continuing education credits (CEUs), which may be necessary for maintaining their certification or renewing their license.

Nurses can learn from subject-matter experts, connect with peers, and discover the newest developments in nursing informatics by attending professional conferences and workshops. On a variety of informatics-related themes, these events include keynote speeches, panel discussions, interactive workshops, and poster presentations.

Informatics professionals from all over the world travel to popular nursing informatics conferences like the American Nursing Informatics Association (ANIA) Annual Conference,

Healthcare Information and Management Systems Society (HIMSS) Conference, and American Medical Informatics Association (AMIA) Annual Symposium.

Nurses can authenticate their nursing informatics knowledge, skills, and competencies through programs for certification and credentialing. These courses provide advanced nursing informatics degrees, certificates, and qualifications that attest to a nurse's skill and dedication to their career.
Nursing informatics professionals can benefit from certification programs like the American Nurses Credentialing Center's Informatics Nursing Certification (RN-BC) and credentials like the Healthcare Information and Management Systems Society's Certified Professional in Healthcare Information and Management Systems (CPHIMS), both of which are offered by the ANCC.

Numerous tutorials, courses, and materials on nursing informatics are available on online learning platforms. These platforms provide nurses freedom and convenience by enabling them to access instructional materials at their own pace and from any location with an internet connection.
Courses in health IT systems, data analytics, telehealth applications, and informatics fundamentals are available on platforms like Coursera, edX, LinkedIn Learning, and Nurse.com. To improve learning, a lot of these self-paced courses have interactive modules, tests, and assessments.

Healthcare environments frequently use informatics tools, systems, and technologies, and specialized training programs offer practical expertise with them. These programs, which can be provided by vendors, consulting firms, or healthcare organizations, might concentrate on certain topics like telehealth integration, CDSS optimization, or EHR deployment.

Nursing educators can enhance their practical skills and competences in nursing informatics by participating in training programs that combine classroom education, practical labs, and real-world simulations. Upon completion of some programs, certification or continuing education credits may also be awarded.

Access to educational resources, networking opportunities, and professional development programs are among the benefits of membership in professional organizations like the American Medical Informatics Association (AMIA), Healthcare Information and Management Systems Society (HIMSS), and American Nursing Informatics Association (ANIA).

Becoming a member of professional organizations gives nurses the chance to network with peers, participate in continuing education and teamwork, and remain up to date on the most recent advancements in nursing informatics.

In order to improve their knowledge, abilities, and competencies in this quickly changing industry, nurses must have access to professional development options in nursing informatics.

Nurses can stay up to date on technological and informatics advancements and further their professional development and career advancement in nursing informatics by taking part in continuing education programs, going to conferences and workshops, obtaining certifications and credentials, and attending specialized training programs.

CHAPTER TWO

Nursing Informatics Theory

A framework for comprehending the function of information technology and information management in nursing practice, education, research, and administration is provided by nursing informatics theory. These theories direct nurses in applying clinical decision-making, evidence-based practice, and patient care through the use of informatics principles. Although there are several nursing informatics theories, Virginia K. Saba and Kathleen A. McCormick's "Competency-Oriented Nursing Informatics Model" is one of the most well-known.

Saba and McCormick created the Competency-Oriented Nursing Informatics Model (CONI) to offer a conceptual framework for comprehending the competences necessary for nursing informatics practice. In order to attain the best possible patient outcomes, the model places a strong emphasis on the integration of nursing science, information management, and technology.

The information, abilities, and theories that support nursing practice are collectively referred to as nursing science, and they form the foundation of the CONI paradigm. By combining data management ideas, technology applications, and informatics principles to improve nursing care delivery, nursing informatics expands on nursing science.

Important informatics competences that are necessary for nursing practice are identified by the CONI model. Information management, technological know-how, clinical decision support, sharing health information, evidence-based practice, leadership, and teamwork are some of these competencies.

The CONI paradigm acknowledges the role that informatics resources and technologies play in assisting nursing practice. Clinical decision support systems (CDSS), telehealth applications, health information exchange (HIE) platforms, electronic health records (EHRs), and data analytics tools are some of these tools.

To support documentation, collaboration, communication, and decision-making in healthcare settings, nurses need to be adept at using these technologies.

The idea of patient-centered care, which highlights the significance of taking patients' unique needs, preferences, and values into account in nursing practice, is fundamental to the CONI paradigm. Nurses may offer individualized, evidence-based treatment that is customized to the particular needs and circumstances of each patient with the use of informatics tools and resources.

The CONI model highlights the value of ongoing education and career advancement while acknowledging the dynamic nature of nursing informatics. To stay current with technological developments and informatics practice, nurses must participate in continual education, training, and skill development. This will help them retain their proficiency in nursing informatics.

A framework for identifying, fostering, and assessing

informatics competencies in nursing practice is offered by the CONI model. To improve their competency in nursing informatics, nurses can utilize the model to pinpoint areas for skill improvement, create learning objectives, and schedule professional development activities.

The CONI model is a useful tool that nursing educators can use to make sure their students are ready to practice nursing informatics after graduation. The model can be modified to fit the requirements of various educational programs and learning situations. It offers nursing students an organized method of teaching informatics concepts, competences, and abilities.

The CONI model can be used by healthcare organizations to evaluate the nursing staff's informatics competencies, pinpoint areas that require development, and create training initiatives to raise nursing informatics competency throughout the institution. Healthcare companies may enhance patient care quality and safety, streamline clinical workflows, and provide better results by investing in the professional development of their nursing informatics personnel.

The CONI paradigm helps nurses use informatics tools and resources to improve clinical practice, advance evidence-based care, and improve patient outcomes by fusing nursing science, informatics principles, technological applications, and patient-centered care.

Theoretical Foundations of Nursing Informatics

The conceptual framework for comprehending the integration of nursing science with information management and technology is provided by the theoretical underpinnings of nursing informatics. The creation, application, and assessment of informatics solutions in nursing practice, education, research, and administration are guided by these principles.

A fundamental idea in nursing informatics, systems theory sees healthcare organizations as complex systems made up of interdependent parts and subsystems. The interconnectedness, interactions, and impact of these elements on the overall behavior of the system are highlighted by this theory.

Systems theory is used in nursing informatics to comprehend how data moves through healthcare institutions, how technology interacts with clinical procedures, and how modifications to one component of the system affect other components. Nurses can find ways to streamline workflow, increase information flow, and improve patient care delivery by using systems thinking.

The design, usability, and efficacy of technological interfaces and computer systems in facilitating human-computer interaction are the main topics of Human-Computer Interaction (HCI) theory. This idea highlights how crucial it is to provide technological solutions that are easy to use, intuitive, and in line with consumers' ergonomic and cognitive needs.

In order to guarantee that clinical decision support systems (CDSS), electronic health record (EHR) systems, and other informatics tools satisfy the needs of end users, such as nurses, clinicians, and patients, HCI theory is applied in nursing informatics. Nurses can improve informatics products' usability, functionality, and satisfaction by putting HCI concepts to use. This will increase user acceptability and adoption.

The theory of Diffusion of Innovations investigates how novel concepts, inventions, and technology are embraced and dispersed within a community. This theory emphasizes important variables, such as social networks, communication channels, organizational context, and perceived innovative features, that affect adoption rates and extent.

The Diffusion of Innovations theory in nursing informatics aids nurses in comprehending the elements that impact the acceptance and application of informatics solutions in healthcare environments. Nurses can successfully incorporate and integrate informatics tools into clinical practice, improving patient care and outcomes by recognizing and proactively addressing adoption hurdles.

The study of information theory focuses on the fundamentals of information transport, communication, and processing inside systems. This theory looks at the encoding, transmission, and decoding of information to provide context and facilitate decision-making.

Information theory serves as the foundation for nursing informatics, guiding the development and application of information systems, data standards, and interoperability frameworks that guarantee precise, prompt, and significant information sharing amongst healthcare settings. Nurses can enhance communication, coordination, and decision-making in patient care by optimizing data capture, documentation, retrieval, and sharing processes through the application of information theory principles.

The theory of Adaptive Structuration looks at how people engage with technology in settings that are organizational. This idea highlights how technology serves as a tool for work completion as well as a social media and organizational tool.

Adaptive Structuration theory is a useful tool in nursing informatics since it helps nurses understand how social structures, norms, and practices inside healthcare organizations shape and are shaped by technology. Nurses can use informatics solutions to improve collaborative work processes, facilitate information exchange, and encourage innovation in healthcare delivery by understanding the interaction between technology and human behavior.

The process of organizational transformation and change is examined by change theory. Initiation, adoption, implementation, institutionalization, and other critical phases of change are identified by this theory, which also looks at the variables that affect effective change management.

Change theory in nursing informatics offers a paradigm for comprehending how to apply informatics solutions—like EHR systems or CDSS—in healthcare organizations in an efficient manner. Nurses can successfully adapt and integrate informatics tools into clinical practice by anticipating resistance to change, including stakeholders, and putting change theory ideas into practice.

The conceptual framework for comprehending the integration of nursing science with information management and technology is provided by the theoretical underpinnings of nursing informatics. Nurses can optimize the design, implementation, and evaluation of informatics solutions to improve patient care, enhance clinical decision-making, and foster innovation in healthcare delivery by applying concepts from systems theory, HCI theory, Diffusion of Innovations theory, information theory, and change theory.

Frameworks for Nursing Informatics Theory

Nursing informatics theory frameworks offer methodical ways to arrange and comprehend the intricate relationships among technology, information management, and nursing practice. These frameworks direct the creation, application, and assessment of nursing informatics solutions, enabling the provision of superior, patient-centered care. Some of the most important frameworks in nursing informatics theory are listed below:

A theoretical framework that investigates the elements influencing people's acceptance and adoption of new technologies is called the Technology Acceptance Model (TAM). According to TAM, people's intentions to utilize technology are significantly influenced by their perceptions of its perceived usefulness and simplicity of use.

TAM can be utilized in nursing informatics to comprehend nurses' attitudes and actions toward informatics systems and instruments. Nurse leaders and educators can create plans to encourage technology use, streamline training, and overcome obstacles by evaluating nurses' opinions of the value and usability of technological solutions.

An expansion of Technology Acceptance Model (TAM) is the Unified Theory of Acceptance and Use of Technology (UTAUT), which incorporates a number of elements impacting technology acceptance, such as performance expectancy, effort expectancy, social influence, and enabling conditions. According to UTAUT, these elements work together to affect users' intended behavior and actual use of technology.

UTAUT offers a thorough framework for comprehending the factors influencing nurses' adoption and usage of technology in the field of nursing informatics. Nurse leaders can create interventions to encourage technology adoption and maximize user satisfaction by taking into account variables like performance expectancy (i.e., perceived benefits of technology), effort expectancy (i.e., perceived ease of use), social influence (i.e., peer and organizational support), and facilitating conditions (i.e., resources and infrastructure).

In four domains—computer abilities, information literacy, informatics knowledge, and informatics skills—the Nursing Informatics Competency Assessment (NICA) model outlines the competences necessary for nursing informatics practice. It was created by Staggers and Thompson. The model offers an organized method for evaluating nurses' informatics proficiency and pinpointing areas in which they should further their careers.

The NICA model is a tool used by nurses, educators, and administrators to assess and improve the informatics competencies of nursing staff. Through the evaluation of nurses' computer abilities, information literacy, informatics knowledge, and informatics skills, organizations can customize training courses and interventions to fit the unique requirements of their staff and advance nursing informatics practice excellence.

A theoretical framework known as the Health Information Technology acceptability Model (HITAM) expands on Technology Acceptance Model (TAM) and highlights the particular elements affecting HIT adoption and acceptability in the healthcare setting. Perceived utility, perceived usability, perceived danger, trust, and organizational support are among the elements that HITAM takes into account.

Within the field of nursing informatics, HITAM offers valuable perspectives on the variables impacting nurses' adoption and utilization of health information technology solutions, including telehealth platforms, clinical decision support systems (CDSS), and electronic health records (EHRs). Nurse leaders can create plans to encourage technology adoption and maximize user satisfaction by taking into account elements including perceived utility, simplicity of use, faith in technology, and organizational support.

A theoretical framework called the Information Systems Success Model (ISSM) looks at the variables that affect how well information systems are implemented in businesses.

Key factors that determine a system's success are identified by ISSM, and these factors include user happiness, system quality, information quality, and individual impact.

When it comes to nursing informatics, ISSM can be used to evaluate how well informatics solutions support nursing practice and help organizations reach their objectives. Nurse leaders can make informed decisions about how best to maximize the success of informatics initiatives by assessing factors like system quality (i.e., usability, reliability), information quality (i.e., accuracy, timeliness), user satisfaction, and individual impact (i.e., productivity, decision-making).

Nursing informatics theory frameworks offer organized methods for comprehending the acceptance, application, and assessment of informatics solutions in nursing practice.

Through the utilization of these frameworks, nurse leaders and educators can appraise nurses' technological attitudes and behaviors, appraise informatics competencies, and maximize the efficacy of informatics endeavors to enhance patient care and results.

Data Collection and Documentation

Nursing practice necessitates data collection and recording as a way for nurses to methodically obtain, document, and share information regarding patient care. In order to support clinical decision-making, facilitate continuity of care, promote patient safety, and maintain regulatory compliance, efficient data collecting and documenting methods are critical.

Nurses can methodically acquire information about a

patient's health status, including physical, psychological, and environmental aspects, through data collection. To evaluate the needs of the patient, pinpoint health issues, and create personalized care plans, this data is employed.

Continuous data gathering helps nurses to assess goal progress, measure the success of interventions, and keep an eye on how a patient's condition develops over time. Clinical decision-making is informed by this data, which also makes it easier to modify the treatment plan as necessary.

The main channel of communication for doctors, therapists, and other allied health professionals within the healthcare team is the data that nurses gather. Ensuring timely and accurate data documentation guarantees that all members of the team can work together to deliver patient care and have access to pertinent information.

Standardized assessment instruments and techniques should be used by nurses to guarantee consistency and dependability in data collecting. Standardized procedures for particular clinical conditions, pain measures, risk assessment instruments, and nursing evaluation forms are a few examples of these tools.

It is the goal of nurses to gather data as completely and precisely as possible, paying close attention to details and recording both objective and subjective observations. Ensuring patient safety and supporting clinical decision-making require accurate and complete data.

Data should be gathered quickly following an assessment or intervention, and information should be promptly documented. Communication and care continuity amongst members of the healthcare team are facilitated by timely documentation, which guarantees that data are accurate and up to date.

Meeting legal and regulatory requirements, such as standards of practice, accreditation requirements, and documentation guidelines established by regulatory bodies like The Joint Commission (TJC) or the Centers for Medicare & Medicaid Services (CMS), depends on accurate and thorough documentation.
Interaction and Care Continuity: A permanent record of patient care actions, evaluations, interventions, and results is provided via documentation. It guarantees continuity of care throughout provider or healthcare environment transfers and gives healthcare practitioners a way to communicate with one another in a variety of contexts.

Research studies, quality improvement programs, and outcome evaluation can all benefit from the data that nurses document. Healthcare organizations can discover areas for improvement, put evidence-based practices into practice, and track the effects of interventions on patient outcomes by looking for trends and patterns in documentation data.

Best Practices for Documentation

Electronic health records, or EHRs, offer a centralized platform for electronically recording patient data, making it easier for healthcare practitioners to access, retrieve, and share information. In addition to following the documentation norms and processes set forth by their company, nurses should be adept users of EHR systems.

In order to guarantee data clarity, consistency, and interoperability, nurses should utilize standardized vocabulary and language in their documentation. Standardized nursing terms that are frequently used are NOC for nursing outcomes, NIC for nursing interventions, and NANDA-I for nursing diagnoses.

Documentation should avoid needless repetition or redundancy and be precise, succinct, and focused on pertinent information. When speaking, nurses should be objective, refrain from using jargon or acronyms that could be confusing, and offer clarification or context when necessary.

When recording patient information, nurses should follow all applicable legal and ethical requirements, including those pertaining to security, privacy, and confidentiality. HIPAA standards should be followed while protecting protected health information (PHI), and nurses should be informed of their organization's policies on patient record access, disclosure, and retention.

Nurses can guarantee the quality, completeness, and integrity of patient information by following best practices for data collection and documentation. This will eventually contribute to safe, efficient, and patient centered care and delivery.

Data Standards and Operability

Nursing informatics relies heavily on data standards and interoperability because they create norms for the gathering, sharing, and application of medical data in a variety of contexts and systems. These guidelines guarantee that data is recorded reliably, consistently, and in a way that various healthcare stakeholders can comprehend and use.The organization, format, and content of healthcare data are governed by established principles, regulations, and specifications known as data standards. In order to facilitate uniform and interoperable data interchange, these standards establish common vocabulary, coding schemes, and data items used in clinical documentation.

Types of Data Standards

Clinical concepts, diagnoses, procedures, drugs, and other healthcare items are described using standardized vocabularies, codes, and classifications defined by terminology standards. A few examples are ICD-10 (International Classification of Diseases), LOINC (Logical Observation Identifiers Names and Codes), and SNOMED CT (Systematized Nomenclature of Medicine - Clinical Terms).

Healthcare systems can transmit electronic messages in a certain format and structure thanks to messaging standards like HL7 (Health Level Seven). Laboratory results, prescription orders, clinical records, and admission-discharge-transfer (ADT) messages are just a few of the healthcare transactions for which HL7 standards define data exchange formats.

Guidelines for the seamless integration and interchange of healthcare data across various systems and organizations are established by interoperability standards. These standards guarantee that data, irrespective of the underlying technology or platform, may be exchanged and comprehended by a wide range of stakeholders.

Advantages of Data Standards

Data standards guarantee that information is recorded, saved, and transferred in a standardized and uniform manner, which promotes interoperability. Interoperable data facilitates data-driven decision-making, care coordination, and collaboration by allowing for smooth sharing and integration across heterogeneous systems.

Data standards offer a uniform framework for recording and classifying healthcare information, which promotes consistency and quality in clinical documentation. Standardized coding schemes and terminologies increase data dependability, correctness, and completeness, which raises the standard of care and aids in clinical decision-making.

Effective data integration and interchange between healthcare systems, applications, and environments are made possible by data standards. Healthcare organizations can enhance care coordination, minimize data fragmentation, and expedite information sharing processes by conforming to uniform standards for data representation and communication.

The capacity of various healthcare systems, apps, and gadgets to communicate and use data in a seamless, accurate, and safe manner is known as interoperability. Healthcare information can be shared, accessed, and used across organizational boundaries because of interoperability, which promotes data-driven decision-making, care coordination, and continuity of care.

Levels of Interoperability

Basic data transmission and reception are made possible by systems' capacity to share data in a standard format and syntax. This is known as foundational interoperability. While data mobility between systems is guaranteed by this degree of interoperability, semantic interoperability—or the capacity to understand and utilize data in a meaningful way—is not.

For data to be correctly understood and interpreted by receiving systems, common data standards and formats must be used. This is known as structural interoperability. This degree of interoperability makes sure that data organization, syntax, and structure are consistent, which makes it easier to integrate and exchange data between different systems.

At the pinnacle of interoperability lies semantic interoperability, which is the capacity to reliably and unambiguously interpret and utilize material that has been transmitted. In order to guarantee that the data are intelligible and therapeutically relevant to users, this degree of interoperability depends on standardized terminologies, vocabularies, and coding systems.

Interoperability makes it possible for healthcare professionals to seamlessly exchange patient data, which facilitates interdisciplinary collaboration, care coordination, and care transitions. Encouraging decision-making and better patient outcomes are facilitated by rapid, accurate, and thorough access to patient data.

Patients are empowered by interoperability to exchange

and access their health information on various healthcare platforms and contexts. Patients can interact with clinicians, take an active role in their care, and make educated decisions about their health with the help of patient portals, personal health records (PHRs), and mobile health apps.

The ability to aggregate, analyze, and share health data among various populations and sources is made possible by interoperability, which aids in population health management programs. Insights into disease patterns, risk factors, and healthcare inequities are provided by integrated data from public health registries, electronic health records (EHRs), and other sources. These insights inform policy decisions and public health actions. Nurses can guarantee that information is properly recorded, documented, and transmitted across varied systems and locations by adhering to standardized terminologies, messaging formats, and interoperability standards. This will eventually improve patient care, safety, and outcomes.

Privacy and data governance

Important components of nursing informatics include data governance and privacy, which center on creating guidelines, protocols, and security measures to guarantee the privacy, security, and integrity of medical records. The framework and procedures for managing and safeguarding data assets are included in data governance, whereas patient privacy refers to the safeguarding of PHI and compliance with legal and ethical requirements.

The management framework and procedures that guarantee the availability, security, quality, and integrity of healthcare data throughout its lifecycle are collectively referred to as data governance. It entails setting up guidelines, norms, roles, duties, and protocols for the efficient and ethical management of data assets. Assigning obligation and duty for managing and preserving data assets inside an organization is known as data stewardship. Data stewards are responsible for monitoring data quality, usage guidelines, access restrictions, and adherence to data governance guidelines.

The creation and use of guidelines, rules, and practices for handling data at every stage of its lifecycle—collection, processing, sharing, and disposal—is referred to as data governance.

Mechanisms for guaranteeing the correctness, consistency, reliability, and completeness of healthcare data are part of data governance. To find and fix data mistakes or discrepancies, quality assurance procedures may include data validation, verification, cleansing, and auditing.

Implementing strong security mechanisms and access controls is part of data governance, which guards against unauthorized access, disclosure, alteration, and destruction of healthcare data. To protect private data and reduce cybersecurity threats, security controls may include audits, authentication, authorization, and encryption.

Data governance is the process of overseeing data from the point of creation to the point of disposal. This involves establishing guidelines for data archiving, disposal, and retention in order to minimize risks and expenses associated with data preservation while maintaining compliance with legal and regulatory requirements.

Benefits of Data Governance

By ensuring the dependability, consistency, and quality of healthcare data, data governance procedures improve the data's usability and credibility for reporting, research, and clinical decision-making.

Healthcare data privacy, security, and confidentiality are governed by legal, regulatory, and industry requirements. Data governance frameworks make sure these criteria are met. Organizations reduce their risk of regulatory infractions and related penalties by following data governance rules and processes.

Standardized data definitions, transparent accountability, and efficient procedures for data gathering, storing, sharing, and analysis are all part of data governance's promotion of efficient management of data assets. Organizations are able to support strategic decision-making activities, increase operational efficiency, and maximize data consumption as a result.

Principles of Privacy

The right of individuals to manage who has access to their personal health information (PHI) and to guarantee its security and confidentiality is known as privacy. In accordance with legal and ethical requirements, healthcare institutions must adhere to privacy principles when collecting, using, disclosing, and protecting PHI.

PHI is only accessed and released by those who are allowed

to do so for proper medical needs, thanks to confidentiality. It is the responsibility of healthcare institutions and providers to protect patient information confidentiality and guard against illegal access or disclosure.

Before collecting, utilizing, or disclosing a patient's PHI for treatment, payment, or healthcare operations, consent principles demand that the patient provide their consent or authorization. Patients are entitled to manage the sharing of their information and to withdraw their consent at any moment.

The idea of data minimization is to simply gather and keep the bare minimum of PHI required for justifiable medical needs. To lower privacy threats, healthcare companies should refrain from collecting or storing sensitive information needlessly and follow data reduction guidelines.

A number of legal and regulatory systems, such as the following, regulate privacy in healthcare:

HIPAA stands for Health Insurance Portability and Accountability Act. HIPAA provides guidelines for healthcare organizations, providers, health plans, and business associates to preserve patient privacy and sets national standards for the privacy, security, and confidentiality of protected health information (PHI).

The HITECH Act, also known as the Health Information Technology for Economic and Clinical Health Act, strengthens enforcement mechanisms and expands HIPAA requirements to include breach notification provisions in order to address security and privacy breaches involving health information exchange (HIE) systems and electronic health records (EHRs).

Regulation on the General Data Protection (GDPR): GDPR sets rules for data protection, privacy, and consent that apply to businesses that handle the personal data of people living in the European Union (EU). When handling patient data from EU citizens, healthcare organizations need to abide with GDPR requirements.

Healthcare personnel are subject to professional codes of conduct and ethical standards that govern how they handle patient information in addition to legal obligations. Maintaining patient confidentiality, upholding patient autonomy, and striking a balance between the right to privacy and the necessity of sharing information to promote public health programs and patient care are examples of ethical considerations.

The growing prevalence of health information exchange (HIE) systems, telehealth platforms, and electronic health records (EHRs) presents significant data governance and privacy risks, such as cybersecurity threats, interoperability problems, and data breaches.

Healthcare companies have difficulties in striking a balance between patient privacy rights and the requirement for data sharing and interoperability. In order to preserve patient confidentiality and avoid illegal access or disclosure, efforts to foster data exchange and collaboration must be balanced with security measures.

Healthcare data security and patient privacy are seriously threatened by the increase in cyberthreats, including ransomware attacks, malware infections, and data breaches. To reduce these risks and protect patient data, healthcare companies need to put strong cybersecurity controls and incident response procedures in place.

Initiatives for health information exchange are designed to make it easier for patients' data to be seamlessly shared among various healthcare systems and organizations. To safeguard patient confidentiality, however, data governance guidelines, encryption standards, and authentication procedures must be followed in order to ensure privacy and security throughout data sharing.

Nursing informatics relies heavily on data governance and privacy to protect the security, confidentiality, and integrity of medical records. Healthcare organizations can protect patient information, uphold trust, and encourage the responsible use of healthcare data for better patient care and outcomes by putting in place strong data governance frameworks, adhering to privacy principles, and meeting legal and regulatory requirements.

CHAPTER THREE

Data Analysis and Decision Making

Nursing informatics, which involves the systematic evaluation and interpretation of healthcare data to enhance clinical practice, improve patient outcomes, and drive organizational decision-making, is fundamentally centered on data analysis and decision-making. Healthcare data can be processed, analyzed, and interpreted using a variety of tools and procedures; on the other hand, decision-making entails applying data-driven insights to guide clinical judgments, interventions, and policy decisions.

Examining, purifying, converting, and analyzing healthcare data to find patterns, trends, connections, and insights that might guide choices and enhance patient care and organizational performance is known as data analysis.

In order to highlight important traits, patterns, and distributions in healthcare data, descriptive analysis entails compiling and displaying the data. Frequency distributions, histograms, and summary statistics (such as mean, median, and mode) are examples of common descriptive approaches. Using a sample of data, inferential analysis entails drawing conclusions or forecasts about the population. Regression analysis, predictive modeling, and hypothesis testing are examples of inferential techniques that are used to find correlations, linkages, or causal effects in the data.

EDA entails examining and displaying data in order to discover patterns, formulate theories, and obtain understanding of underlying structures or relationships. EDA methods include box plots, scatter plots, and correlation analysis to discover meaningful patterns in the data.

Using statistical and machine learning techniques, predictive analytics makes predictions about future trends or events by analyzing past data. Using patterns and correlations found in the data, predictive models can be used to identify individuals who are at-risk, forecast the course of a disease, or improve treatment strategies.

Tools and Techniques

Regression analysis, statistical testing, and predictive modeling are frequently carried out on healthcare data using statistical software tools including SPSS, SAS, R, and Python. Nurses can generate interactive charts, graphs, and dashboards using data visualization tools like Tableau, Power BI, and R Shiny to visually convey patterns and insights in healthcare data.

Large datasets can be analyzed using machine learning techniques, such as classification, clustering, and regression algorithms, to find patterns and generate predictions or suggestions based on the
data available.

In nursing informatics, decisions are made based on clinical knowledge, data-driven insights, and evidence-based practice guidelines. The goal is to make well-informed decisions, interventions, and choices that maximize patient outcomes, raise the standard of care, and improve organizational performance.

Data analysis is essential to Evidence Based Data(EBP)since it provides empirical support, study findings, and data on clinical outcomes to guide clinical interventions and decision-making. In order to direct nurse practice, EBP guidelines and procedures incorporate patient preferences, professional knowledge, and the best available research.

Clinical Decision Support Systems (CDSS): CDSS use clinical data and evidence-based guidelines to give physicians alerts, recommendations, and real-time clinical decision support at the point of treatment. Nurses using CDSS might find possible prescription errors, poor drug responses, or clinical interventions based on patient specific data.

By pointing out areas for improvement, comparing performance measures, and assessing how interventions affect patient outcomes, data analysis supports quality improvement programs. Data-driven insights are used by quality improvement programs to optimize workflows, promote organizational transformation, and improve care delivery.

Data analysis is used in population health management programs to pinpoint interventions, identify patient populations at high risk, and track population-level health results. Across a range of patient populations, data-driven initiatives like risk stratification, care coordination, and preventative interventions seek to enhance health outcomes and lower healthcare costs.

Before collecting, using, or disclosing a patient's health information for clinical or research purposes, nurses must get the patient's informed consent. With informed permission, patients can make independent decisions about their health information and are guaranteed to understand the goal, risks, and advantages of data collection.

Protecting the privacy and confidentiality of patient health information is a moral and legal duty for nurses. Access restrictions, encryption technologies, and data security procedures protect patient data against abuse, unauthorized access, and disclosure.

Through the monitoring of performance measures, the facilitation of data-driven decision-making, and the identification of practice improvement opportunities, clinical decision support systems assist ongoing efforts to improve quality.

CDS systems help healthcare organizations evaluate the effectiveness of interventions, pinpoint areas for improvement, and hone decision support algorithms to better serve the requirements of physicians and patients by evaluating usage statistics, clinical outcomes, and adherence to recommendations.

By giving physicians prompt access to evidence-based information, assisting with clinical decision-making, and encouraging adherence to best practices and clinical guidelines, clinical decision support is essential to the advancement of evidence-based practice. Healthcare organizations can improve clinical outcomes, promote patient safety, and provide high-quality, patient-centered care in a variety of healthcare settings by utilizing CDS systems to integrate evidence into clinical workflows.

Quality Improvement and Patient Safety

In order to maximize patient outcomes, improve treatment

processes, and reduce risks of harm, quality improvement (QI) and patient safety programs are crucial parts of healthcare delivery. While patient safety stresses eliminating errors, adverse events, and injury to patients, quality improvement focuses on methodically evaluating, monitoring, and improving healthcare procedures and results.

Data-driven methods are used in patient safety and quality improvement programs to track performance indicators, identify areas for improvement, and keep an eye on patient outcomes.
To find trends, patterns, and chances for action, healthcare organizations gather and examine data from a variety of sources, such as electronic health records (EHRs), incident reporting systems, and patient feedback.

Root cause analyses (RCAs) are used in quality improvement and patient safety initiatives to look into adverse events, near misses, and other patient safety occurrences.
RCAs help establish corrective actions and preventive measures by identifying underlying issues, such as communication breakdowns, system failures, or human factors, that contribute to errors or undesirable outcomes.

The implementation of standardized procedures, clinical guidelines, and best practices is encouraged by quality improvement initiatives to guarantee safety, dependability, and consistency in the provision of healthcare.
In order to enhance adherence to best practices, decrease variability, and direct clinical practice, physicians can benefit from the clear recommendations and decision support tools that evidence-based guidelines and protocols offer.

To measure progress and pinpoint opportunities for improvement, patient safety, performance metrics, and safety indicators are continuously monitored as part of quality improvement and patient safety initiatives.
Frequent feedback systems that promote open communication, shared learning, and accountability among healthcare teams include safety huddles, peer review, and morbidity and mortality conferences.

Initiatives aimed at improving patient safety and quality must involve interdisciplinary teamwork and involvement at all organizational, departmental, and team levels in the healthcare system.
Together, clinicians, administrators, quality improvement specialists, and patient advocates create and put into practice plans aimed at streamlining care delivery, cutting down on hazards, and strengthening patient safety culture.Human factors and ergonomics concepts are integrated into patient safety and quality improvement initiatives to provide safer medical technology, workflows, and systems.

Leadership Roles in Nursing Informatics

Leadership positions in nursing informatics cover a broad spectrum of duties with the goals of spearheading strategic plans, encouraging creativity, and maximizing the application of data and technology in nursing practice and healthcare provision. To promote change, encourage the uptake of technological solutions, and enhance patient outcomes, these leadership positions necessitate a blend of clinical experience, informatics understanding, and leadership abilities.

The Chief Nursing Informatics Officer(CNIO)

Within healthcare organizations, the CNIO is a senior leadership role tasked with providing strategic direction, vision, and oversight for nursing informatics efforts.

In order to create informatics strategies, set investment priorities, and match technological solutions with organizational objectives and priorities, CNIOs work in conjunction with executive teams, IT departments, and nursing leadership.

CNIOs support the integration of technology and data-driven techniques into nursing practice and patient care, advance a culture of innovation and continuous improvement, and champion nursing informatics as a strategic goal.

Nurse Informaticist Specialist

Expert practitioners with superior knowledge and abilities in data analytics, nursing informatics, and healthcare technology are known as nurse informaticist specialists.

They are essential to the deployment, personalization, and enhancement of clinical decision support systems, electronic health record (EHR) systems, and other informatics solutions.

Working with interdisciplinary teams, nurse informaticist professionals assess workflows, create system configurations, and create best practices for data management, clinical decision-making, and documentation.

Nurse Informatics Manager/Specialist

The daily management of nursing informatics projects and programs within healthcare institutions is the responsibility of nurse informatics managers or coordinators.

They oversee groups of informatics nurses and support personnel, plan project operations, and guarantee that they are in line with the objectives and priorities of the company. Policies, procedures, and standards for nursing informatics practice, documentation, and data management are developed in collaboration with IT departments, nursing leadership, and other stakeholders by nurse informatics managers.

Clinical Informatics Specialist

Clinical informatics specialists assist in the installation, optimization, and use of technological solutions in clinical practice. They are front-line clinicians with specialized training in nursing informatics.

Nursing staff receives instruction, education, and support on clinical decision support technologies, electronic health record (EHR) systems, and other informatics applications from them.

Clinical informatics specialists act as a point of contact between nursing staff and IT departments, promoting user demands, resolving problems with workflow, and assisting interdisciplinary teams in their communication and cooperation.

Nursing Informatics Educator

Nurse informatics educators create and administer educational curricula, instructional materials, and competence evaluations to assist nursing personnel in gaining informatics expertise.

They create curricula, instructional modules, and practical workshops on subjects like clinical decision support, telemedicine, EHR documentation, and data management.

To encourage informatics capabilities and lifelong learning among nursing practitioners, nursing informatics educators work in partnership with academic institutions, professional groups, and continuing education providers.

Telehealth Nurse Informaticist

Telehealth nurse informaticists are experts in using communication and technology to monitor patient health, conduct virtual consultations, and provide nursing care from a distance.

They work together with multidisciplinary teams to create telehealth processes, procedures, and guidelines while making sure that best practices and legal requirements are followed.

Nurse informaticists specializing in telehealth offer nursing staff education, training, and assistance about telehealth technologies, remote patient monitoring devices, and virtual care delivery models.

Research and Innovation Leader

To enhance the science and practice of nursing informatics, research, pilot projects, and innovation efforts are carried out by nursing informatics leaders in research and innovation roles.

They work together with educational institutions, research centers, and business associates to plan studies, gather and process data, and communicate results that support evidence-based practice and stimulate innovation in nursing informatics.

Leaders in research and innovation help create new technologies, informatics solutions, and care delivery models that enhance clinical workflows, improve patient outcomes, and advance the efficacy and efficiency of nursing practice.

Leadership positions in nursing informatics are varied and complex, including management, clinical, instructional, and research duties. Leaders in nursing informatics are essential to advancing the nursing profession by fostering innovation, advancing best practices, and maximizing the use of technology and data to improve patient care outcomes and clinical processes. Nursing informatics professionals promote nursing practice in an increasingly digital and data-driven healthcare environment by transforming healthcare delivery and advocating for patients through their knowledge, advocacy, and teamwork with interdisciplinary teams.

CHAPTER FOUR

Change Management and Decision Making

In the healthcare industry, "change management" refers to the methodical process of organizing, coordinating, and overseeing organizational changes in order to streamline workflows, raise standards of care, and improve patient outcomes. Organizational reorganization, process enhancements, policy updates, technology developments, and process improvements are all commonplace in healthcare businesses. In order to successfully navigate these changes and minimize opposition, maximize adoption, and guarantee the sustainability of gains, it is imperative to employ effective change management practices.

A clear vision for the ideal future state and a strong commitment from the leadership are necessary for change projects. Promoting change, motivating stakeholders, and cultivating an environment that values innovation and ongoing development are all tasks that leaders must perform expertly.

Gaining buy-in, creating support, and addressing issues during the change process all depend on engaging stakeholders, who include frontline personnel, clinicians, patients, and other important stakeholders. A sense of accountability and ownership among stakeholders is fostered by effective communication and collaboration, which raises the possibility of successful change adoption.

Analyzing present procedures, defining goals and objectives, and determining the need for change all require careful planning and assessment.Organizations might benefit from using change management frameworks, like the ADKAR model (Awareness, Desire, Knowledge, Ability, Reinforcement), to plan and carry out change projects in a methodical manner.

Throughout the transition process, it is imperative to maintain open and honest communication in order to manage expectations, answer queries, and keep stakeholders informed. To guarantee that communications are understandable, timely, and pertinent, communication channels should be customized to the requirements and preferences of various stakeholders.

It is vital to furnish personnel with sufficient training and assistance to foster proficiency, self-assurance, and openness towards embracing novel procedures or technologies. Training programs must to be customized to meet the unique requirements of end users, including practical experience, job assistance, and continuous support to promote learning and skill development.

Finding areas for improvement and evaluating the success of change projects depend on gathering input from stakeholders and keeping an eye on developments. Organizations are better equipped to modify tactics, remove obstacles, and maintain gains over time when they engage in ongoing assessment.

The process of managing change starts with determining the need for change. Then, a change management plan is developed, present procedures are evaluated, and stakeholders are analyzed. This plan describes the change initiative's goals, objectives, schedules, communication tactics, and resource needs.

Organizations carry out the change plan during the phase of implementation which includes staff training, the introduction of new procedures or technology, and progress monitoring. To encourage adoption and get past opposition to change, leadership support, stakeholder participation, and effective communication are essential.

Organizations track developments, gather input, and assess how change initiatives are affecting important performance indicators including staff productivity, patient happiness, and quality of service. To maximize change outcomes, strategies, tactics, and interventions are modified based on evaluation findings.

New procedures or habits must be continuously supported, integrated into company culture and practices, and reinforced in order for change to be sustained. To maintain the momentum of change and avoid reverting to earlier procedures, organizations must foster a culture of continuous improvement, celebrate accomplishments, and acknowledge the efforts of employees.

Healthcare organizations frequently experience resistance to change because of things like uncertainty anxiety, a sense of losing one's independence, and worries about adding more work or upsetting workflows. Proactive communication, engaging stakeholders, and addressing issues with empathy and honesty are all necessary to overcome opposition.

Change management initiatives may face difficulties due to a lack of staff, funds, and time. To optimize the impact of change initiatives, organizations need to set priorities for their resources, set aside money for support and training, and make the most of their current alliances and expertise.

Healthcare systems frequently have a number of interconnected procedures, numerous stakeholders, and regulatory requirements. In order to guarantee that objectives and resources are in line, managing change in such settings calls for meticulous planning, coordination, and cooperation amongst various stakeholders.

The implementation of novel technologies, including clinical decision support systems, electronic health records (EHRs), or telehealth platforms, might present difficulties because of interoperability problems, technical complexity, and the requirement for staff training. To maximize the benefits of technology adoption, organizations need to invest in strong IT infrastructure, intuitive user interfaces, and extensive training programs.

Driving innovation, improvement, and transformation in healthcare businesses requires effective change management. Healthcare executives may successfully manage change, involve stakeholders, and create long-term gains in the standard of care, patient outcomes, and organizational performance by adhering to fundamental concepts, procedures, and tactics.

Electronic Health Record Implementation

The process of implementing an electronic health record (EHR) is intricate and entails switching from paper-based record-keeping to digital technologies for patient health information management. EHRs have many advantages, such as better care coordination, easier access to data, and more efficiency in the provision of healthcare. To guarantee

EHR system uptake and optimization, however, thorough planning, stakeholder involvement, and continuing support are necessary for a successful implementation.

Important Stages for EHR Setup:

Evaluation and Planning: Perform an exhaustive evaluation of the objectives, requirements, and preparedness of the organization for the deployment of the EHR.
Establish the project's goals, parameters, and schedule for implementation.
Invite important parties to participate in the planning process, such as patients, IT workers, administrative staff, and clinicians.

Selecting a Vendor:
Consider factors such vendor reputation, affordability, usability, interoperability, and system functionality while evaluating EHR providers.
To make sure that the selection process is in line with organizational needs and preferences, ask for proposals, organize demos, and involve stakeholders.

Customization and Configuration: Tailor the EHR system to the unique clinical requirements, workflows, and preferences of the company.
Establish order sets, templates, and decision support guidelines to aid in clinical recording and decision-making.
Assure compatibility with current systems and incorporate other data sources, like pharmacies and labs.

Instruction and Training: Give employees thorough instruction and training on EHR features, workflows, and best practices.

To meet user demands and encourage system proficiency, provide ongoing assistance, online tutorials, and hands-on training sessions.

Programs for training should be customized to meet the requirements and preferences of various user groups, including as IT workers, nurses, administrators, and physicians.

Go-Live and Transition: To find and fix any problems or concerns, thoroughly test and validate the EHR system before to going live.

Adopt a staged go-live strategy, launching pilot programs in select departments or units before extending to the full company.

During the changeover phase, offer on-site assistance and troubleshooting to reduce interruptions and ensure a smooth transition into the new system.

Optimization and Continuous Improvement: To pinpoint areas for optimization and improvement, track system performance, user input, and key performance indicators (KPIs) on a regular basis.

Get input from interested parties and apply user suggestions to updates and improvements to the system.

Apply patches, upgrades, and updates on a regular basis to guarantee system security, functionality, and legal compliance.

Major adjustments to organizational culture, workflows, and procedures are necessary while implementing EHRs. The effective adoption and optimization of the EHR system depend on controlling opposition to change, resolving workflow interruptions, and guaranteeing stakeholder buy-in.

Careful preparation and validation are necessary to guarantee the correctness, completeness, and integrity of data while transferring information from paper records or outdated systems to the new EHR system. If not properly addressed, data migration issues like duplicate records, incorrect data mapping, and data loss can have an adverse effect on patient care and safety.

For seamless care coordination and information exchange, it is imperative to achieve interoperability with external systems and communicate data with laboratories, other healthcare providers, and health information exchanges (HIEs). In order to overcome interoperability obstacles including mismatched data formats, data standards, and technological impediments, cooperation and standardization initiatives must be made throughout the healthcare ecosystem.

To ensure that EHR adoption and proficiency are effective, it is imperative to provide workers with sufficient training and support. Tailored training programs, continuous education, and easily accessible support resources are necessary to address the diverse skill levels, learning styles, and training requirements of various user groups. When implementing an EHR, it is critical to safeguard patient health information against unauthorized access, disclosure, or breaches. Encryption, access limits, strong security measures, and auditing systems are some of the ways that sensitive data can be protected and HIPAA and other regulatory compliance can be guaranteed. Maximizing productivity,

efficiency, and user satisfaction inside the EHR system requires simplifying and optimizing procedures.
The system's usability and acceptance can be increased by tailoring templates, order sets, and clinical decision support tools to the preferences and workflows of clinicians.

The primary goals of healthcare management are to increase patient happiness, care quality, and efficiency. Two crucial components of this process are workflow analysis and optimization. Workflow optimization is the process of finding areas for improvement and putting those ideas into practice in order to improve organizational performance and streamline workflows. Workflow analysis is the methodical examination of the order of tasks, processes, and interactions involved in providing healthcare services.The system's usability and acceptance can be increased by tailoring templates, order sets, and clinical decision support tools to the preferences and workflows of clinicians.

Key Principles of Workflow Analysis

Understanding and recording present processes, including activities, responsibilities, handoffs, and decision points, is the initial step in workflow analysis. Interviewing employees, watching operations in action, and going over paperwork like policies, protocols, and standard operating procedures can all be part of this.

The steps, inputs, outputs, and decision points of a process are shown and documented using workflow diagrams, also known as flowcharts or process maps. Workflow mapping makes it easier to spot inefficiencies, bottlenecks, and redundancies as well as areas that could use improvement.

Workflow diagrams and stakeholder input analysis are valuable tools for locating process bottlenecks, gaps, and pain spots that could affect patient outcomes, quality, or efficiency. Errors, rework, delays, and failures in communication are common complaints.

Workflow variability can lead to inefficiencies and irregularities in the provision of care. Examples of this include variations in practice patterns, preferences, and resource availability. Standardizing procedures and enhancing predictability and dependability need an understanding of and response to workflow variability.

Simplifying and standardizing procedures to get rid of pointless stages, duplicate steps, and delays is known as streamlining. Redesigning workflows, automating tedious chores, and allocating resources optimally are a few ways to reduce inefficiencies and increase productivity.

Improving coordination and communication across departments, stakeholders, and members of the care team is crucial to the efficient operation of the workflow. Collaboration and timely information transmission can be facilitated by putting communication tools like messaging apps, multidisciplinary huddles, and electronic health records (EHRs) into use.

Utilizing technological solutions can simplify procedures, cut down on manual labor, and enhance data accessibility and accuracy. Examples of these solutions include workflow management software, telemedicine platforms, and clinical decision support systems. Investing in technology solutions that are easy to use and customized to meet end users' wants and preferences is essential for successful adoption and optimization.

Standardizing procedures, policies, and best practices contributes to ensuring safety, quality, and consistency in the provision of healthcare. Creating order sets, care pathways, and protocols based on the best available research and clinical recommendations encourages adherence to standard operating procedures and lowers process variability.

Successful implementation and adoption of improved procedures, standards, and technological solutions require staff education and training. Providing personnel with thorough training programs, practical workshops, and continuous assistance fosters competence, confidence, and readiness to accept change and improve processes.

Reduced inefficiencies and streamlined processes result in quicker throughput, reduced wait times, and more output. Staff members can concentrate on value-added activities, such providing direct patient care, instead of administrative work or pointless stages, thanks to optimized workflows.

The uniformity, dependability, and safety of care delivery are increased by standardizing procedures, lowering variability, and putting evidence-based practices into practice. Workflows that are optimized reduce errors, stop unfavorable things from happening, and enhance patient outcomes.

Quick care delivery, simplified procedures, and effective workflows all add to a satisfying patient experience. Patient satisfaction and system involvement are increased by reducing wait times, enhancing communication, and offering integrated treatment.

Workflows that are optimized save waste, money spent, and resources, which benefits healthcare companies financially. Financial performance and operational efficiency are raised through streamlining procedures, getting rid of duplication, and raising productivity.

Providing employees with standardized procedures, user-friendly technology solutions, and effective workflows boosts engagement, morale, and job satisfaction. Increased retention rates and less burnout are the results of staff members feeling respected, supported, and prepared to provide high-quality care.

In the healthcare industry, workflow analysis and optimization are critical tactics for raising productivity, standards of care, and patient outcomes. Through methodical analysis of existing procedures, identification of areas for enhancement, and implementation of modifications to optimize workflows, healthcare establishments can increase their operational efficiency, curtail expenses, and provide superior, patient-focused medical care.

CHAPTER FIVE

Usability and User Experience Design

When developing and implementing healthcare technologies, such as electronic health records (EHRs), clinical decision support systems (CDSS), and mobile health applications, usability and user experience (UX) design are crucial factors to take into account. While UX design focuses on providing pleasant and meaningful experiences for users by taking into account their wants, preferences, and goals, usability refers to a system's efficiency and simplicity of use. Ensuring UX design and usability is crucial in the healthcare industry to boost clinician satisfaction, encourage adoption, and improve patient care.

Key Principles of Usability

The system should be simple enough for users to pick up and use right away, without requiring a lot of training or prior knowledge. Users may learn and adopt products more easily when they have intuitive design, clear instructions, and guided tutorials.

Systems that are easy to use allow users to complete activities quickly and achieve their objectives with the least amount of time and effort. Shortcuts, logical navigation, and streamlined processes increase user productivity and lower cognitive burden.

After extended periods of non-use, users ought to be able to recall how to operate the system. Learning and memory retention are supported and reinforced by visual clues, familiar terminology, and consistent design patterns.

With the use of features for error prevention, clear feedback, and warnings, usable systems reduce the likelihood of errors. Error messages ought to be clear, concise, and useful in order to aid users in learning from their mistakes and preventing them in the future.

User pleasure and perceived usefulness are strongly correlated with usability. Positive user experiences and long-term engagement and loyalty are fostered by systems that are simple to use, engaging, and match user needs.

Key Principles of User Experience (UX) Design

Understanding user needs, objectives, and preferences is the first step in UX design. Designers may better understand people and develop solutions that fulfill their requirements and expectations by conducting user research, developing personas, and conducting usability testing.

UX designers concentrate on developing aesthetically pleasing user interfaces and simple interactions that draw users in and facilitate their jobs. Clear layout, responsive design, and consistent branding improve usability and strengthen brand identity.

Information is arranged and structured by UX designers in a logical, user-friendly, and navigable manner. Users can locate information more quickly and effectively with the aid of contextual signals, clear labeling, and hierarchical menus.

Users with disabilities or impairments are taken into account in UX design, along with their varied demands and talents. Regardless of their physical or mental capabilities, all users may access, navigate, and interact with the system efficiently because to accessibility-focused design.

Iterative user experience design entails testing prototypes, getting user feedback, and making adjustments to designs based on observations and insights. Iteration and continuous improvement support designers in recognizing and resolving usability problems as they optimize the user experience over time.

Advantages of UX and Usability Design in Medical Technology

Healthcare technologies that are easy to use and well-designed have a higher chance of being accepted and utilized by users. Good user experiences drive engagement and encourage system usage over time, improving patient and provider outcomes.

Healthcare technology usability problems and design defects can have detrimental effects on patient safety. Error avoidance techniques, intuitive workflows, and clear interface design minimize the chance of user mistakes and unfavorable outcomes.

Clinicians can work more quickly and effectively with usable technologies, which saves time and lessens the administrative load. Increased efficiency frees up doctors to spend more time directly caring for patients and less time figuring out intricate workflows or systems.

At the point of care, clinical decision support systems (CDSS) with a well-designed interface give doctors access to timely, pertinent, and useful information. Effective CDSS tools facilitate better decision-making, increase diagnostic precision, and improve patient outcomes for physicians.

Health technologies that are patient-centered and easy to use enhance the patient experience. Patient-friendly mobile apps, telehealth platforms, and patient portals enable people to take an active role in their care, interact with healthcare providers, and easily obtain health information.

Healthcare organizations may increase adoption, improve patient care, and more by putting the needs of their users first, creating user-friendly interfaces, and improving the user experience.and encourage the pleasure of clinicians. All phases of the development lifecycle should use usability and UX design concepts to provide solutions that satisfy user needs and improve outcomes for patients and providers.

The Role of the Nurse Informaticist

The nurse informaticist has a dynamic and diverse role in healthcare delivery, utilizing a broad variety of duties to optimize the utilization of data management systems and information technology. In order to improve patient care outcomes, streamline clinical workflows, and advance evidence-based practice, nurse informaticists span the gap between nursing practice, technology, and data science.

It takes continual education, training, and assistance to ensure that nurses are proficient, competent, and confident while integrating technology into their practice.
Informatics proficiency, technological literacy, and practical experience with EHRs, CDSS, telemedicine, and other medical technologies are all incorporated into nursing school programs.
Nurses can stay up to date on developing technologies, best

practices, and regulatory requirements for incorporating technology into nursing practice through continuing education seminars, workshops, and simulation exercises.

Aligning technology with user demands, organizational priorities, and clinical procedures is essential for its successful integration into nursing practice.
Nurses work in conjunction with informaticists, IT departments, and interdisciplinary teams to optimize system usability, configure workflows, and design technology solutions.

The utilization of technology to enhance efficiency, efficacy, and patient happiness in nursing practice is made possible via workflow analysis, user input, and continuous improvement initiatives.
When it comes to using technology to improve communication, expedite workflows, and give patients more control over their care, nurses are essential. By means of education, training, and cooperation with interdisciplinary teams, nurses may effectively utilize technology to enhance nursing practice and provide superior, patient-focused care in a variety of healthcare environments.

Using Evidence-based Practice and Clinical Decision Support

At the point of care, clinical decision support (CDS) systems are computer-based instruments that help medical personnel make well-informed clinical decisions by offering pertinent patient-specific data, evidence-based guidelines, and practical recommendations. By incorporating clinical expertise, industry best practices, and research information into the decision-making process, these systems are essential to the advancement of evidence-based practice (EBP).

Clinical decision support systems facilitate the simple retrieval of research findings, clinical protocols, and evidence-based guidelines for particular patient situations or scenarios by healthcare practitioners.
Instead of depending only on clinical judgment or gut feeling, CDS systems enable doctors to make well-informed judgments by using the most recent data from reliable sources and medical literature.

CDS systems provide recommendations, alerts, and reminders that are customized to each patient's requirements and preferences by analyzing patient data, including test results, diagnostic results, and medical history, in real-time.
These recommendations, which assist physicians in identifying relevant interventions, diagnostic tests, and treatment options that are in accordance with current best practices, are based on evidence-based guidelines, clinical pathways, and decision support rules.
Clinical decision support systems offer clinical algorithms, risk assessment calculators, and decision support tools to help physicians diagnose illnesses, choose the best courses of action, and track patients' progress.
Clinicians can assess patient risk factors, forecast outcomes, and personalize treatment strategies to maximize positive patient outcomes and reduce negative occurrences with the use of CDS systems, which use predictive models and

evidence-based algorithms.

At the point of care, CDS systems provide physicians with real-time warnings, reminders, and suggestions to encourage adherence to clinical guidelines and evidence-based procedures.
These notifications, which assist physicians in adhering to established protocols and enhancing patient safety and quality of care, may include medication warnings for drug interactions or allergies, immunization or screening reminders, and prompts for evidence-based therapies or clinical pathways.

Clinical decision support systems provide informed consent and collaborative care planning by offering evidence-based information, treatment alternatives, and risk assessments to support shared decision-making between physicians and patients.Through patient involvement in the decision-making process and the clear and understandable presentation of information, CDS systems enable patients to take an active role in their care, make well-informed decisions, and work toward common treatment objectives.

It has been demonstrated that incorporating clinical decision support into clinical workflows increases patient safety, promotes adherence to evidence-based practices, and lowers healthcare costs by lowering variability in the provision of care.
In a variety of healthcare settings and patient populations, studies have shown how beneficial CDS systems are in lowering prescription mistakes, averting adverse events, and enhancing adherence to therapeutic standards.

Through the monitoring of performance measures, the facilitation of data-driven decision-making, and the identification of practice improvement opportunities, clinical decision support systems assist ongoing efforts to improve quality.

CDS systems help healthcare organizations evaluate the effectiveness of interventions, pinpoint areas for improvement, and hone decision support algorithms to better serve the requirements of physicians and patients by evaluating usage statistics, clinical outcomes, and adherence to recommendations.

By giving physicians prompt access to evidence-based information, assisting with clinical decision-making, and encouraging adherence to best practices and clinical guidelines, clinical decision support is essential to the advancement of evidence-based practice. Healthcare organizations can improve clinical outcomes, promote patient safety, and provide high-quality, patient-centered care in a variety of healthcare settings by utilizing CDS systems to integrate evidence into clinical workflows.

Healthcare IT strategic planning

Creating a thorough road map to direct the adoption, execution, and optimization of information technology (IT) solutions in support of corporate priorities and goals is known as strategic planning for healthcare IT. Efficient strategic planning guarantees congruence between information technology endeavors and the broader mission, vision, and goals of the healthcare establishment. One could plan by doing the following actions.

Analyze the internal and external environments in-depth to find possibilities, problems, and new developments affecting healthcare IT.

Evaluate the competencies, resources, strengths, and weaknesses of the company in addition to external elements like market trends, legal needs, and technology developments.

Establish the organization's strategic priorities, goals, and objectives for its IT projects related to healthcare.

Sync IT objectives with overarching corporate priorities, such boosting operational effectiveness, fostering financial sustainability, and improving patient care results.

Involve important stakeholders in the strategic planning process, such as IT personnel, administrators, physicians, patients, and outside partners.

To make sure that IT efforts fit stakeholders' needs, preferences, and expectations, get their opinions, suggestions, and comments.

Create a strategic IT plan outlining the organization's technology-leveraging goals, objectives, and strategies in order to accomplish strategic priorities.

Establish the parameters for IT initiatives, including their timetable, resources, and scope. Also specify the key performance indicators (KPIs) that will be used to gauge their success.

Sort IT projects into priority lists according to how well they support organizational objectives, how they might affect patient care and operations, and how practical they are to implement.

When prioritizing efforts, take into account variables like cost, complexity, and risk, and distribute resources appropriately.

Examine the systems, capabilities, and IT infrastructure in place to find any weaknesses and potential opportunities for development.
Based on their functionality, compatibility, scalability, and alignment with corporate needs and goals, evaluate technology options, vendors, and solutions.

For any IT project, create a thorough implementation strategy that includes deadlines, goals, roles, and resource distributions.
Establish project governance frameworks, roles, and communication procedures to guarantee efficient stakeholder coordination and cooperation.

Provide an effective change management plan to help employees and stakeholders embrace IT efforts.
To guarantee that end users are competent in utilizing new systems and technologies efficiently, offer thorough training and assistance.

Provide systems for tracking and assessing how IT projects are doing in relation to the objectives and results of the organization.
To determine areas for development and to evaluate the efficacy and efficiency of IT solutions, monitor KPIs, performance metrics, and user input on a regular basis.

Encourage a culture of constant growth by asking for input,

taking lessons from accomplishments and setbacks, and making necessary adjustments to plans and methods.

To be competitive in the changing healthcare landscape and to keep ahead of industry trends, promote innovation and investigation of emerging technologies.

Healthcare strategic planning IT is necessary to provide excellent outcomes for patients and stakeholders, maximize the value of IT projects, and match technology expenditures with organizational goals. By including stakeholders, outlining precise goals and objectives, setting priorities for projects, putting strong governance and

Healthcare companies can create and carry out strategic IT strategies that support their long-term success, mission, and vision by implementing change management methods.

CHAPTER SIX

Health informatics policy and regulation

In the field of healthcare informatics, policy and regulation are essential for directing the creation, application, and use of IT systems that guarantee patient security, privacy, and high-quality care. Standards, norms, and requirements are set forth by policies and laws for a variety of topics, including data security, interoperability, telehealth, health information exchange (HIE), and the usage of electronic health records (EHRs).

A complicated regulatory structure, comprising national, state, and international laws as well as industry standards and recommendations, governs healthcare informatics.

The Department of Health and Human Services (HHS), the Office of the National Coordinator for Health Information Technology (ONC), the Food and Drug Administration (FDA), and the Centers for Medicare & Medicaid Services (CMS) are important regulatory bodies and agencies that are involved in healthcare informatics.

The Health Insurance Portability and Accountability Act (HIPAA) lays out criteria for the use and disclosure of protected health information (PHI) by covered entities and business associates, as well as standards for the security and privacy of PHI.

Enacted as part of the American Recovery and Reinvestment Act (ARRA) of 2009, the Health Information Technology for Economic and Clinical Health (HITECH) Act fortifies HIPAA privacy and security provisions while extending enforcement powers and stiffening penalties for noncompliance.

The Meaningful Use program, commonly known as the Medicare and Medicaid EHR Incentive Programs, offers financial rewards and penalties to qualified healthcare organizations and providers who implement and demonstrate the meaningful use of certified EHR technology.

To guarantee compatibility, functionality, and security, the ONC Health IT Certification Program sets requirements and standards for EHR technology certification.

In order to encourage interoperability and make it easier for patients, payers, and healthcare providers to exchange health information, the 21st Century Cures Act was passed in 2016.

The concepts, rules, and conditions for the safe and interoperable exchange of health information between networks and organizations are established by the ONC's Trusted Exchange Framework and Common Agreement (TEFCA).

States, jurisdictions, professional associations, payers, and state medical boards define the requirements for practice, licensure, and payment for telehealth and telemedicine.

In response to the COVID-19 epidemic, state and federal governments have loosened regulations and granted temporary waivers in order to increase access to telehealth services, ease limitations on licensure and reimbursement, and encourage the provision of virtual care.

Clinical terminologies, messaging formats, and data exchange protocols are just a few of the standards and specifications for the interchange of health information that are established by the ONC's Standards and Interoperability Framework.

The Fast Healthcare Interoperability Resources (FHIR) standard, created by HL7 International, makes use of contemporary web-based APIs and data formats to facilitate the transmission of electronic health information.

Regulations and industry standards for cybersecurity and data protection are applicable to healthcare businesses in order to protect patient information and guard against cyberattacks, unauthorized access, and breaches.

Encryption, risk management, access controls, and incident response are all governed by regulations like the Health Information Technology Cybersecurity Certification Program (HIT-Cyber) and the HIPAA Security Rule.

Institutional Review Board (IRB) requirements, ethical principles, and data sharing rules to ensure the protection of human subjects, privacy, and confidentiality are among the laws and regulations controlling healthcare informatics research and innovation.

The Department of Health and Human Services (HHS) established the Common Rule, which lays forth guidelines for protecting human subjects in research that is funded by or carried out by federal agencies.

In healthcare informatics, policies and regulations play a crucial role in safeguarding patient privacy, guaranteeing data security, fostering interoperability, and propelling the uptake of technological solutions that enhance patient outcomes.

To reduce risks and guarantee compliance with relevant laws and regulations, healthcare businesses need to employ strong compliance programs, follow industry standards and best practices, and stay up to date on regulatory requirements. Working together, stakeholders such as legislators, regulators, medical professionals, technology companies, and patient advocates may better address new issues, foster innovation, and advance the use of informatics to change the way healthcare is delivered.

Professional Duty and Ethics

Healthcare professionals, particularly those in the informatics area, are guided in their conduct and decision-making by core concepts of ethics and professional accountability. Respecting professional obligations and ethical norms is crucial in the field of nursing informatics in order to safeguard patient confidentiality, foster confidence, and guarantee the moral application of data and technology.

Protecting patient privacy and confidentiality requires nurses and informaticists to uphold ethical and legal obligations by preventing illegal access, use, or disclosure of sensitive health information.

Nurses must make ensuring that patient data is handled, stored, and sent securely in order to comply with privacy laws like HIPAA. This applies to patient data stored in electronic health records (EHRs), health information exchanges (HIE), and telehealth platforms.

Before collecting, using, or disclosing a patient's health information for informatics purposes, nurses and informaticists must get valid informed consent in order to respect the patient's right to autonomy and informed decision-making.

Informatics systems ought to facilitate patients' access to their medical records, provide them with the tools to decide how best to use their data, and provide them the authority to take part in joint decision-making over their care.

By making sure that data entered into informatics systems is correct, full, and up to date, nurses and informaticists are accountable for preserving the integrity and accuracy of health data.

Following best practices, documentation standards, and quality assurance procedures helps avoid mistakes, inconsistencies, and misunderstandings that might jeopardize patient safety and care quality.

It is the professional duty of nurses and informaticists to promote inclusive and equitable practices in order to address gaps in healthcare technology access and use.

In order to guarantee that informatics treatments are both accessible and sensitive to the varied needs of patient groups, it is imperative that variables like digital literacy, language hurdles, cultural preferences, and socioeconomic position be taken into account.

Organizational policies, professional standards, and ethical guidelines governing the use of data and technology in healthcare practice must be followed by nurses and informaticists.

A few examples of ethical issues in the planning, execution, and assessment of informatics interventions are guaranteeing data security, honoring patient choices on the sharing and use of their data, preventing conflicts of interest, and maintaining professional integrity.

When it comes to using informatics tools and technologies, nurses and informaticists are responsible for their choices and actions. This includes considering how their choices may affect patient care outcomes, organizational performance, and ethical standards.

Open communication regarding the goals, advantages, drawbacks, and restrictions of informatics interventions—as well as any possible conflicts of interest or prejudices—with patients, coworkers, and other stakeholders is a key component of transparency in informatics practices.

It is the professional duty of nurses and informaticists to pursue continual education, skill building, and competency enhancement in order to stay current with developments in healthcare technology and informatics practice.

Nurses and informaticists can uphold high standards of practice and ethical integrity in their work by participating in professional organizations, continuing education, and adhering to professional rules of conduct and ethics.

New Developments and Technologies

New developments in healthcare informatics and technology are changing the way healthcare is delivered, increasing patient outcomes, streamlining clinical processes, and completely changing how healthcare is accessible and provided. Artificial intelligence (AI), machine learning, blockchain, Internet of Things (IoT), genomics, and virtual reality (VR) are just a few examples of the many solutions that these technologies cover.

Healthcare is undergoing a revolution thanks to artificial intelligence (AI) and machine learning technologies, which allow computers to analyze massive amounts of data, spot trends, and forecast outcomes to aid in diagnosis, treatment planning, and clinical decision-making.

Predictive analytics, image recognition, natural language processing, and personalized medicine are a few of the AI applications in healthcare that enable healthcare practitioners to give more accurate, efficient, and timely care.

Using video conferencing, smartphone apps, wearable technology, and Internet of Things sensors, telehealth and remote monitoring technologies allow patients to access virtual care, consultations, and monitoring services from a distance.

Telehealth solutions lessen the workload for medical facilities and physicians while increasing patient engagement, increasing access to care, and improving care coordination, especially for underprivileged or rural populations.

Blockchain technology makes it possible to store, share, and manage health data in a transparent, safe, and decentralized manner. This makes it easier for healthcare systems to manage patient consent, interoperability, and data interchange.

Blockchain-based solutions facilitate patient autonomy over access to their health information, improve data security, integrity, and privacy, and expedite administrative tasks including revenue cycle management and claims processing.

Smartwatches, activity trackers, and medical sensors are examples of wearables and Internet of Things (IoT) devices that offer continuous monitoring of vital signs, activity levels, and health indicators. These devices also provide real-time data for tailored health management and remote patient monitoring.
IoT solutions enable patients to take charge of their health and well-being by supporting proactive interventions, early detection of health changes, and self-management techniques.

By evaluating a person's genetic composition, lifestyle factors, and biomarkers, precision medicine and genomics are enabling tailored approaches to healthcare that customize preventive, diagnosis, and treatment plans to each individual's specific needs.
Understanding disease risk, treatment response, and therapeutic efficacy through genetic sequencing, pharmacogenomics, and precision oncology enables more focused and efficient interventions as well as better patient outcomes.

Healthcare facilities are using VR and AR technologies for patient education, training, simulation, and immersive therapy experiences.
In a risk-free virtual environment, VR simulations allow medical professionals to hone their clinical skills, practice difficult procedures, and improve patient safety. On the

other hand, AR superimposes digital data onto the real world to help with patient education, surgical navigation, and medical imaging.

In healthcare settings, robotics and automation technologies are assisting clinical workflows, improving surgical precision, and automating repetitive operations.

Minimally invasive operations, fewer surgical errors, and better patient outcomes are made possible by surgical robots, and administrative work, data input, and workflow automation are streamlined by robotic process automation (RPA) to boost productivity and cut expenses.

Healthcare companies may now examine enormous information, spot trends, and forecast results to guide clinical decisions and resource allocation thanks to advanced data analytics and predictive modeling tools like machine learning algorithms and predictive analytics.

In order to improve health outcomes and lower healthcare costs, predictive models for disease surveillance, patient risk stratification, and population health management enable proactive treatments, early detection of health trends, and targeted therapies.

Unprecedented improvements in patient care, clinical practice, and healthcare delivery are being fueled by new technology and developments in healthcare informatics. Healthcare organizations can increase clinical results, optimize resource use, improve patient experience, and improve access to care by utilizing these technologies.

To fully realize the potential of emerging technologies in healthcare informatics and ensure their ethical and equitable use in promoting everyone's health and well-being, it is imperative to address issues pertaining to data privacy, interoperability, regulatory compliance, and workforce readiness.

Artificial Intelligence and Predictive Analysis

In healthcare informatics, predictive analysis and artificial intelligence (AI) are two potent instruments that transform clinical decision-making, improve patient outcomes, and expedite the delivery of healthcare. In order to forecast future occurrences or results, predictive analysis entails examining both past and current data to find patterns, trends, and connections. Conversely, artificial intelligence (AI) describes how computers, usually computer systems, simulate human cognitive processes so they may carry out tasks that would generally need human intellect, including education, logic, solving problems, and making decisions.

Advanced statistical models, machine learning algorithms, and data mining approaches are utilized in predictive analysis in the healthcare industry to examine various sources of healthcare data such as genomics, medical imaging, electronic health records (EHRs), and clinical data.
In order to find patterns, correlations, and risk variables linked to particular outcomes—like disease initiation, progression, treatment response, readmission rates, and patient outcomes—predictive models are trained using historical data.
Healthcare providers can use predictive analysis to prioritize interventions, identify high-risk patients, stratify patient populations, and customize treatment approaches based on predicted insights and individual risk profiles.

Natural language processing (NLP), machine learning, deep learning, computer vision, robotics, and cognitive computing are just a few of the many uses of AI technology in healthcare.

NLP makes it possible for computers to recognize, comprehend, and produce human language, which is useful for voice recognition, chatbots, virtual assistants, clinical documentation, and other applications.

Large datasets are analyzed by machine learning algorithms, which then use the patterns they find to forecast outcomes and automate decision-making processes related to diagnosis, prognosis, treatment planning, and drug discovery.

Deep learning models, which draw inspiration from the anatomy and physiology of the human brain, are particularly good at handling unstructured data, including text, signals, and medical pictures. These models have also demonstrated potential in areas including disease classification, pathology detection, and medical imaging analysis.

Artificial intelligence (AI) and predictive analysis are closely related fields. Predictive models rely heavily on AI algorithms to improve their complexity, scalability, and accuracy.

In predictive analysis, artificial intelligence (AI) techniques including neural networks, random forests, support vector machines, and ensemble methods are frequently used to analyze complicated datasets, extract insightful information, and produce predictions that can be put into practice.

Healthcare companies may fully utilize their data assets,

uncover hidden patterns and linkages, and obtain predictive insights to guide clinical decision-making, enhance patient outcomes, and optimize resource allocation by integrating AI and predictive analysis.

Numerous applications of AI and predictive analysis are found in healthcare informatics, such as risk stratification, population health management, clinical decision support, disease prediction, personalized treatment, and operational efficiency.
Forecasting disease outbreaks, identifying individuals at risk of acquiring chronic diseases, predicting readmissions to hospitals, optimizing treatment regimens, and anticipating the demand for healthcare resources are all possible with predictive models.
Clinical decision support systems driven by artificial intelligence (AI) evaluate patient data, medical literature, and clinical guidelines to deliver evidence-based advice, warnings, and reminders to healthcare professionals at the point of care, enhancing patient safety, treatment efficacy, and diagnosis accuracy.

Predictive analysis and artificial intelligence (AI) combined provide many advantages, such as better patient safety, tailored care, cost savings, and increased clinical results.
To guarantee the moral and responsible application of AI and predictive analysis in healthcare, however, issues including data quality, interoperability, bias, openness, privacy, and regulatory compliance need to be resolved.
Artificial intelligence and predictive analysis are potent instruments with great potential to improve patient care, revolutionize healthcare delivery, and advance medical

practice. Healthcare organizations can maximize the potential of their data assets, spur innovation, and enhance population and individual health outcomes by utilizing the synergies between AI and predictive analysis.

However, in order to fully exploit the transformative potential of AI and predictive analysis in healthcare informatics, issues with data governance, ethics, privacy, and equity must be resolved.

CHAPTER SEVEN

Patient Engagement and Empowerment

The term "patient engagement" describes how actively people participate in their healthcare journey, including making decisions about their own care, voicing their questions and concerns, and working with medical professionals to accomplish common treatment objectives.
Patients who are engaged in their care are well-informed, driven, and equipped to take charge of their health, follow their treatment regimens, and actively engage in health promotion and preventative initiatives.
Patient education, collaborative decision-making, training healthcare personnel in communication techniques, providing access to health information and resources, and utilizing technology-enabled solutions like patient portals and mobile health applications are some of the tactics used to encourage patient engagement.

Encouraging patients to take charge of their health, make educated decisions, and speak up for their own needs in terms of care is known as patient empowerment.
Patients who are empowered possess the information, abilities, self-assurance, and independence necessary to actively engage in healthcare decision-making, voice their preferences and values, and work together as partners in their treatment with healthcare providers.
Through information, encouragement, and support,

empowerment initiatives work to increase patients' sense of self-efficacy, health literacy, communication skills, and capacity for self-management.

Numerous advantages are linked to patient empowerment and involvement, such as better treatment adherence, lower healthcare costs, more patient happiness, and more efficient use of available resources.

Patients who feel empowered and involved are more likely to follow their doctors' instructions, make good lifestyle choices, and actively manage long-term illnesses, all of which improve disease control and reduce the risk of complications.

Patient-centered care delivery, enhanced communication, shared decision-making, and a more cooperative and trustworthy relationship between patients and healthcare professionals are all facilitated by patient empowerment and involvement.

Techniques for Encouraging Patient Empowerment and Engagement

Give patients access to pertinent, clear, and reliable health information so they can decide for themselves what medical care and health issues to pursue.

Provide options to patients, go over the advantages and disadvantages with them, and take into account their preferences, values, and objectives when making treatment decisions. Encourage patients and healthcare professionals to communicate in an honest, open, and transparent manner by paying attention to the patients' worries, answering their inquiries, and including them in the planning of their care.

Utilize technology-enabled resources to help people manage their health whenever and wherever they are by facilitating communication, providing access to health information, and enabling remote monitoring through patient portals, mobile health apps, and telehealth platforms.

Give patients the tools, resources, and emotional support they need to access community services, understand the healthcare system, and speak up for their own medical needs.

Notwithstanding the advantages of patient empowerment and engagement, patients may find it difficult to actively participate in their care due to issues like technology constraints, cultural and socioeconomic inequities, and impediments to health literacy.

In order to overcome these obstacles, healthcare institutions must implement patient-centered, culturally aware strategies, offer specialized assistance and education, and guarantee that all patients have equal access to medical resources and technology.

In order to encourage active participation, teamwork, and shared decision-making between patients and healthcare providers, patient empowerment and engagement are essential components of patient-centered care. Healthcare organizations may improve health outcomes, increase patient happiness, and foster a culture of patient-centeredness and empowerment by giving patients the tools they need to take charge of their health, make educated decisions, and actively participate in their treatment.

Views from around the world on nursing informatics

Global viewpoints on nursing informatics cover a wide range of issues, difficulties, and possibilities pertaining to the acceptance, application, and use of information and communication technologies (ICT) in nursing practice and the provision of healthcare globally. Nurses are essential in using technology to improve patient care outcomes, streamline clinical workflows, and address healthcare issues. Nursing informatics is becoming more and more recognized as a vital component of healthcare systems worldwide.

Electronic health records (EHRs), health information exchange (HIE), telemedicine, and other ICT solutions are being adopted by healthcare systems worldwide more and more in order to facilitate evidence-based practice, increase care coordination, and improve access to care.

However, the rate at which health information technology are adopted and integrated differs throughout nations and regions, depending on variables including infrastructure, financial resources, legal and cultural standards.

For nurses to effectively use ICT solutions in their practice and contribute to the global progress of nursing informatics, nursing informatics education programs and competencies are crucial.

Nursing schools and professional associations are essential in creating and advancing informatics competencies, curricula, and certification programs that guarantee nurses have the skills, knowledge, and mindset necessary to succeed in a healthcare setting that is becoming more and more digital and data-driven.

As healthcare systems work to facilitate seamless sharing and exchange of patient information across organizational boundaries, geographic regions, and healthcare settings, interoperability and health information exchange are crucial challenges in nursing informatics globally.

To guarantee that ICT systems are interoperable and to make it easier for patients, healthcare providers, and other stakeholders to share health information, standardized terminologies, data exchange protocols, and interoperability frameworks are crucial.

Globally, telehealth and remote care delivery are becoming more and more significant parts of nursing practice, especially in underserved and rural areas where access to healthcare services may be limited.
Through the use of wearable technology, smartphone apps, and video conferencing, telehealth solutions allow nurses to provide virtual care, consultations, and monitoring services remotely. This improves patient outcomes, increases access to treatment, and improves care coordination.

Across the globe, data security, privacy, and ethical issues are critical to nursing informatics as healthcare companies work to safeguard patient data, preserve privacy, and respect moral principles when utilizing ICT solutions.
To secure patient privacy and preserve public confidence in healthcare systems, adherence to data protection laws, ethical standards, and best practices for data security—such as encryption, access controls, and audit trails—is crucial.
In order to address shared opportunities and challenges and advance nursing informatics globally, cooperation and information sharing among nations and regions are crucial.

Nursing informatics professionals worldwide can

collaborate, network, and share knowledge through global health informatics initiatives like the International Medical Informatics Association (IMIA) and the Nursing Informatics Special Interest Group (NI-SIG). This promotes the creation and sharing of nursing informatics standards, best practices, and innovations.

The adoption, implementation, and utilization of nursing informatics solutions are greatly influenced by socioeconomic and cultural issues on a worldwide scale. Inequalities in healthcare resources, digital literacy, and technological access have a bearing on healthcare outcomes and equity.

It is imperative to tackle socioeconomic and cultural barriers by means of focused interventions, community involvement, and culturally aware methodologies to guarantee fair distribution of nursing informatics solutions and enhance health outcomes for all groups.

The significance of utilizing information and communication technology to improve nursing practice, patient care outcomes, and global healthcare concerns is underscored by global perspectives on nursing informatics. Nursing informatics professionals can advance nursing practice and the provision of high-quality, patient-centered care globally by fostering interoperability, developing nursing informatics competencies, addressing data security and privacy concerns, and encouraging collaboration and knowledge exchange among stakeholders.

GLOSSARY OF TERMS

Nursing informatics: A specialization that manages and disseminates knowledge, data, and information in nursing practice by fusing computer science, information science, and nursing science.

Electronic Health Record(EHR): An electronic version of a patient's paper chart that includes test results, immunization records, treatment plans, diagnoses, prescriptions, and other healthcare data.

Health information technology, or HIT, is the use of technology for electronic health record keeping, management, and exchange. It includes telehealth, mobile health (mHealth), health information exchange (HIE), and electronic health records (EHRs).

Clinical Decision Support Systems (or CDSS) are software programs that give medical practitioners access to patient-specific data and clinical knowledge to help with diagnosis, treatment planning, clinical decision-making, and patient management.

Interoperability is the capacity of various devices, apps, and information systems to communicate, understand, and use data without difficulty across corporate borders and in healthcare settings.

Telehealth refers to the practice of providing healthcare remotely through the use of digital technologies and telecommunications. This includes telemedicine, telepsychiatry, virtual consultations, and remote monitoring.

Health Information Exchange (HIE): The electronic exchange of health-related data between healthcare practitioners, organizations, and patients throughout various geographic locations and healthcare systems.

Patient portals are safe, secure online spaces where patients may get their medical records, get in touch with doctors, make appointments, get medication refills, and take part in telehealth visits.

Artificial Intelligence is the simulation of human intelligence processes by computers to carry out activities that ordinarily require human intelligence.Machine learning, natural language processing, computer vision, and robotics are examples of artificial intelligence (AI).

Predictive analytics is the process of analyzing past and current data to find patterns, trends, and relationships in order to forecast future occurrences or results. It makes use of statistical algorithms and machine learning techniques.

Clinical workflow is the order in which healthcare professionals carry out their duties, procedures, and activities in order to provide patient care. This includes assessment, diagnosis, treatment, documentation, and follow-up.

Data governance refers to the structure, guidelines, procedures, and controls that guarantee the security, confidentiality, and integrity of medical data at every stage of its lifecycle, including gathering, storing, using, and exchanging it.

Usability: The degree to which healthcare information systems, apps, and gadgets are simple, efficient, and enjoyable for users to interact with and traverse in order to complete tasks and reach objectives.

Change management is an organized method of managing the people, procedures, and technologies involved in implementing changes to workflows, healthcare information systems, and practices in order to accomplish desired results and reduce opposition.

Population health management include risk assessment, care coordination, preventive treatments, and health promotion. It is the proactive management of a specific population's health outcomes and healthcare demands.

Clinical documentation is the process of documenting patient interactions, evaluations, diagnoses, courses of treatment, and results in medical records, such as discharge summaries, progress notes, nursing assessments, and care plans.

Data security is the process of preventing unauthorized use, disclosure, change, or destruction of medical records by putting security mechanisms like authentication, access controls, and encryption in place.

Healthcare analytics is the process of examining and evaluating data related to healthcare in order to find patterns, gauge performance, and provide useful information for clinical, operational, and financial decision-making.

Quality Improvement: Using data-driven initiatives and evidence-based practices, quality improvement is a systematic strategy to continuously monitor, evaluate, and improve the safety and quality of healthcare services, processes, and results.

Patient safety is the process of preventing mistakes, unfavorable outcomes, and patient injury while providing healthcare services by putting safety precautions, guidelines, and best practices into place.

www.ingramcontent.com/pod-product-compliance
Lightning Source LLC
Chambersburg PA
CBHW050316230526
45471CB00005B/2217